MULTIMODAL TREATMENT OF ACUTE PSYCHIATRIC ILLNESS

Multimodal Treatment of Acute Psychiatric Illness

A GUIDE FOR HOSPITAL DIVERSION

*Justin M. Simpson and
Glendon L. Moriarty*

COLUMBIA UNIVERSITY PRESS   NEW YORK

COLUMBIA UNIVERSITY PRESS
Publishers Since 1893
New York   Chichester, West Sussex

cup.columbia.edu
Copyright © 2014 Columbia University Press

Library of Congress Cataloging-in-Publication Data

Simpson, Justin M.
   Multimodal treatment of acute psychiatric illness : a guide for hospital diversion /
Justin M. Simpson, Glendon L. Moriarity.
      p. ; cm.
   Includes bibliographical references and index.
ISBN 978-0-231-15882-4 (cloth : alk. paper) — ISBN 978-0-231-15883-1 (pbk. : alk. paper) —
ISBN 978-0-231-53609-7 (ebook)
   I. Moriarty, Glendon.   II. Title.
   [DNLM: 1. Mental Disorders—therapy. 2. Acute Disease—therapy.
3. Community Mental Health Services. 4. Crisis Intervention. WM 400]

   RC455
   RC480.6—DC23

                                                                        2013016128

Columbia University Press books are printed on permanent and durable acid-free paper.
This book is printed on paper with recycled content.
Printed in the United States of America

C 10 9 8 7 6 5 4 3 2 1
P 10 9 8 7 6 5 4 3 2 1

Cover design by Milenda Nan Ok Lee
Cover art © Getty Images

References to websites (URLs) were accurate at the time of writing.
Neither the author nor Columbia University Press is responsible for URLs
that may have expired or changed since the manuscript was prepared.

TO THE MANY PEOPLE ON THE PATH TO RECOVERY FROM MENTAL ILLNESS,
AND TO THOSE WHO WISH TO HELP THEM ON THEIR JOURNEY

CONTENTS

A 43-YEAR-OLD WOMAN with a history of bipolar disorder and multiple episodes of inpatient treatment has recently experienced an increase in the severity of her symptoms. Her mood is unstable, and she reports feeling "out of control." Recent financial difficulties have caused intense feelings of despair accompanied by thoughts that life is not worth living. She has had some success with medication, but nothing has controlled her symptoms for a substantial period of time. Her husband is discouraged because of the frequent trips to the hospital, continuous contact with emergency services and law enforcement, and constant worry that his wife is going to hurt either herself or someone else. She recently began participating in an assertive community treatment program, and her treatment team knows that if they do not effectively stabilize her, she will have to return to the hospital yet again, even though neither she nor her family wants this.

DILEMMA

The number of Americans with severe mental illness is estimated to be 6 percent of the population. When applied to the 2010 U.S. Census population estimate for ages 18 and older, this figure translates to approximately fourteen million people (U.S. Census Bureau, 2011a). Many of these individuals require periodic inpatient treatment to achieve mental health stability and to function normally. Unfortunately, being displaced from the community even for a short period of time might result in the loss of employment, housing, social supports, and other important aspects of life.

Hospitalization is not the only option for individuals with severe mental illness who experience episodes of psychiatric instability. Community-based alternatives to inpatient care have been available for decades. There are a variety of hospital diversion programs currently available around the country. These programs, including assertive community treatment (ACT), mobile crisis home treatment (MCHT), crisis stabilization, and partial hospitalization are preferred by consumers and are generally more cost effective than inpatient psychiatric care (Ruggeri et al., 2006; Ligon & Thyer, 2000; Granello, Granello, & Lee, 1999; Essock, Frisman, & Kontos, 1998).

Hospital diversion programs are assigned the task of helping individuals, such as the woman described above, manage their symptoms and cope with adversity in the least restrictive environment. However, inpatient treatment is often unnecessarily the first choice in the effort to stabilize a person experiencing an acute phase of his or her particular illness. In many cases inpatient hospitalization occurs because the service providers working within hospital diversion programs have not been trained in helping clients who are decompensating or in crisis (Hunter et al., 2009; Young et al., 2000; Chinman et al., 1999).

There has been a push by government bodies, consumer advocacy groups, and managed care agencies to decrease state psychiatric hospital beds around the country over the past decade (Lipton, 2001), even though the need for those beds remains high. For instance, in Virginia—a state that has shut down psychiatric hospitals and continues to reduce beds in existing ones—recently passed legislation that makes even more people eligible for involuntary commitment to a psychiatric hospital (Virginia DMHMRSAS, 2008). The predicament is obvious; there are fewer hospital beds and more people who will require a bed. As a solution, Virginia is creating more community-based programs, such as assertive community treatment and crisis stabilization, to support individuals in an acute stage of mental illness. Workers within these programs need to develop competency in acute psychiatric care in order to best help consumers.

OVERVIEW

This book offers readers both a conceptual framework and a practical guide for providing brief stabilizing mental health treatment to individuals with severe mental illness. The initial chapters present a theoretical and structural base from which the reader can implement treatment strategies. This section of the text includes an overview of hospital diversion programs, integrated and multimodal treatment, the treatment of severe mental illness, and brief and crisis intervention.

The practical component of the text consists of an integrated and systematic set of interventions that are designed to bring psychiatric stabilization to individuals with severe mental illness (i.e., those with schizophrenia or schizoaffective disorder, bipolar or major depressive disorder, severe anxiety, or substance dependence) who are experiencing mental health decompensation, an emotional or psychological crisis, relapse of substance use, or a mood or psychotic episode. Within a guiding framework, consisting of four intervention phases, specific treatment strategies tailored to certain diagnoses are provided in a step-by-step manner. The treatment approach is considered integrative and multimodal because it includes several empirically supported therapeutic tools that are derived from various clinical orientations and targets multiple aspects of the client's life.

Acute psychiatric illness is the phrase used in the title of this text to describe the condition for which the treatment protocols are targeted. Other terms that have a similar meaning include mental health decompensation, psychological crisis, behavior crisis, and psychotic, anxiety, or mood episode. For the purposes of this book, acute psychiatric illness can be defined as a period in which a person's ability to cope with various stressors or natural condition-related symptom fluctuations has been unsuccessful and the result includes significant impairment in daily functioning, severe emotional disturbance, or behavioral problems.

THE UNIQUE BENEFITS OF THIS BOOK

Because it is not feasible to rely on hospitalization for severely mentally ill individuals who decompensate, the interventions that are offered in the hospital have to be provided by service providers involved in community-based programs. This book helps to bridge the gap between the clinical resources that are used in the psychiatric hospital and other psychiatric or psychological settings and the community-based programs that are often more oriented toward case management. The book can assist crisis stabilization, assertive community treatment, and other acute care program staff in forming accurate conceptualizations, developing appropriate treatment plans, and providing effective interventions for clients served.

This work is distinctive because it

- provides a standardized guide for conducting stabilizing interventions that service providers across disciplines and education levels can use;
- offers a theoretical and research base from which to conceptualize acute care needs and related interventions;
- describes specific intervention strategies in the context of hospital diversion programs;
- focuses primarily on crisis or acute care with the severely mentally ill; and
- provides the reader a step-by-step protocol that is diagnosis specific instead of vague guidelines.

Finally, as the information offered here helps mental health service providers to be efficient and effective, the clients served will be less likely to be displaced from their home or suffer other adverse consequences. Still, in addition to quality-of-life benefits, there are cost benefits that could result from a decrease in the utilization of general hospitals, regional and state psychiatric hospitals, and jails by individuals with severe mental illness (Latimer, Bond, & Drake, 2011; Latimer, 2005, 1999; Kamis-Gould et al., 1999). Among secondary benefits is the possibility that employee turnover may decrease as service providers become more competent in making effective decisions, which will lead to less burnout.

FOCUS ON HOSPITAL DIVERSION PROGRAMS

There are many different treatment settings and service programs through which mentally ill individuals are treated. There are also a large number of programs that specifically target individuals who are at risk for hospitalization or inpatient treatment (e.g., intensive case management, intensive outpatient treatment, and day programs or partial hospitalization). An attempt to develop an intervention manual that is relevant to each of the unique programs is too daunting of a task for such a manual would likely fail to be significantly relevant to any one program. Therefore a smaller group of mental health service programs—hospital diversion programs— has been chosen as the target audience of this text. The text is most relevant to assertive community treatment, mobile-crisis, crisis stabilization, and partial hospitalization programs.

HOW TO USE THIS BOOK

The book is designed to be user friendly, but a few points might facilitate the clinician's ability to begin using it immediately. First, an effort was made to separate the actual intervention components from the theoretical and conceptual information. Consequently once clinicians have become familiar with the multimodal acute care approach in general, they can turn right to the intervention information, simply matching the diagnosis or presenting problem of the client with the appropriate chapter. They can then begin using the tools provided.

In general clinicians will want to begin with the assessment phase and then move to the other three phases in order. It is not necessary, however, to follow the order of interventions within each phase. Certainly there will be instances where clinicians might only use one or two of the interventions, and this is appropriate. Several strategies are provided so that clinicians can find something that works for each client who presents with various needs. In some settings there will not be enough time or resources to implement all the strategies described. For instance, some programs do not have the ability to conduct drug testing. Also, center-based programs might not be able to address social and environmental issues as easily as home-based programs can.

It is important that treatment providers refrain from using techniques that are beyond their training level or degree of competence. To help clinicians determine which techniques require a higher level of clinical competence, an intervention difficulty guide that includes beginner, intermediate, and advanced difficulty levels was created. The guide is discussed in depth in chapter 5 and other chapters.

Many well-established hospital diversion programs have demonstrated success at decreasing the need for psychiatric hospitalization, but there is also evidence of a need for improved crisis intervention and effective clinical care. This book will improve programs by increasing the treatment teams' ability to effectively stabilize individuals in crisis. Furthermore, it can be used as a training resource for those who are new to the mental health field.

The ultimate goal is to provide quality care to the large population of individuals with severe mental illness. The information presented is intended to ensure that such individuals receive appropriate care during the times they are most vulnerable. It is a difficult but rewarding task to help reduce the suffering of these courageous people who may battle horrific symptoms and devastating losses throughout a large portion of their lives. For individuals who experience severe mental illness, the road to recovery often involves multiple challenges and occasional crises. Those who have committed themselves as helpers must be fully prepared when called on in times of need.

Disclaimer: No one should engage in the practice of mental health care, including the interventions described in this text, without proper training and supervision. The authors are not liable for misuse of this text.

MULTIMODAL TREATMENT OF ACUTE PSYCHIATRIC ILLNESS

1

Hospital Diversion Programs

THE EFFORT TO BRING MENTALLY ILL PERSONS out of institutions and back into the community began a number of years ago. The Community Mental Health Centers Act of 1963 was created to provide for community-based care as an alternative to institutionalization, and the process of deinstitutionalization has continued at varying levels since then (Grob, 2008). The current trend has resulted in the development of several alternatives to inpatient treatment. The goal of these programs is to stabilize in the community, and preferably in their own home, individuals who are experiencing crisis.

There is evidence to suggest hospital diversion programs will continue to grow and play a stronger role in treating severe mental illness (SMI). First, the need for effective hospital diversion and crisis stabilization programs has been a focal point of political discourse over the past few years. Virginia, like Tennessee (Tennessee, 2007) and North Carolina (North Carolina Dept. of Health and Human Services, 2005), is making significant shifts in community mental health:

> [The] governor . . . announced today plans for restructuring Virginia's mental health care system. The comprehensive plan redirects resources into programs that provide more community-based care for people with mental illness allowing them to receive treatment closer to their homes, families, and friends. . . . The community system must be enhanced to provide a "safety net" for consumers in short term-crisis. (Commonwealth of Virginia, 2001)

Second, the literature in the areas of hospital diversion and community-based mental health services is consistently growing. For instance, a peer-reviewed article search using the PsycINFO and Academic Search Premiere databases produces approximately six hundred hits for "assertive community treatment"; half of these articles were published after 2002. Third, there appears to be a consensus among researchers that it is typically more beneficial for an individual experiencing acute mental illness to receive community-based care (Ruggeri et al., 2006; Ligon & Thyer, 2000; Granello, Granello, & Lee, 1999; Warner, 1995; Merson et al., 1992).

WHY DO HOSPITAL DIVERSION PROGRAMS EXIST?

Hospital diversion or intensive community treatment programs exist for several reasons. One reason is that they can cut down on the high costs of inpatient treatment. Acute psychiatric illness episodes create financial hardships for mentally ill individuals and society in general because of both treatment costs and lost employment (Kessler et al., 2008). Another reason is that less invasive interventions, such as treatment through hospital diversion programs, are generally preferred by clients because they typically do not have to leave their home for lengthy periods of time or suffer other unnecessary disruptions in their life (Ben-Porath, Peterson, & Piskur, 2004; Ruggeri et al., 2006).

Hospital diversion programs also exist because there are simply not enough hospital beds for the large number of individuals who become mentally unstable. In the United States there was an 88 percent reduction in psychiatric hospital beds between 1955 (339 beds per 100,000 population) and 1994 (40 beds per 100,000 population) (Szmuckler & Holloway, 2001). This decline in available beds has occurred because of deinstitutionalization, which was prompted by a variety of legal, financial, advocacy, and other issues (Torrey, 1997). Unfortunately deinstitutionalization has caused an increase in the number of chronically mentally ill persons who are homeless or in jail (Lamb, 2001; Torrey, 1997).

A National Institute of Mental Health (NIMH) panel summarized the negative consequences of deinstitutionalization and the climate in which hospital diversion programs were born as follows:

> The institutionalization of severely mentally ill people, particularly in hospital back wards, constituted a form of societal paternalism in which many

persons suffered bleak, meaningless lives. With deinstitutionalization and the lack of a community support system, many former patients and others with severe mental illnesses have been given nearly absolute individual liberty but at a very high price. Now that patients can be committed to treatment services only if they are extremely and imminently dangerous to themselves or society, our society allows individuals incapable of realistic planning to struggle through life and wander the streets. Like ships without rudders, homeless people with severe mental illness are free, but at significant risk to life and without much hope of happiness. (Attkisson et al., 1992)

The current state of mental health care is not as bleak because several community supports are now in place. However, there is room for substantial growth.

Legal cases such as *L. C. and E. W.* v. *Olmstead*, in which two female patients who no longer needed inpatient care were not discharged because of a lack of community program availability, prompted the United States Supreme Court to rule that individuals must be treated by way of community-based programs whenever possible (Heath, 2005). Various economic and political influences have also facilitated the growth of community-based care for individuals with mental illness. Advances in pharmacology, advocacy movements involving groups like the National Alliance on Mental Illness (NAMI), and state and federal budget crises are among these influences (Menikoff, 1999a).

Hospital diversion programs are frequently used to help individuals transition from an inpatient setting to the community, as this can be a very difficult period of time. Many times these individuals are not fully stabilized (Bruchner & Yoon, 2009; Kaliski, 1997). Also, those who have been hospitalized for extended periods may become accustomed to or dependent on constant care and attention and may have difficulty readjusting to community life (Hocking, Phare, & Wilson, 2005; Proehl, 1938). In many cases the individual might not receive professional follow-up care for weeks following discharge from the hospital (Predictors, 2007). Because of these challenges, there is an increased risk of relapse, decompensation, and suicide attempts or other problematic behaviors (Torrey, 1997).

The use of hospital diversion programs is essential to every community. The many benefits include decreased mental health care costs as costly hospital visits are avoided, and increased safety for all persons in the community as mentally ill persons are treated before their condition leads to illegal activities. These programs not only benefit communities as a whole; more important, they often produce significant improvement in functioning and life satisfaction for their consumers. Lamb (2001:5) writes, "In the community, most of these [chronically mentally ill] patients can have something very precious—their liberty, to the extent that they can handle it. Furthermore, if we provide the resources, they can realize their potential to attain some of life's milestones."

Another reason these programs are necessary is their ability to relieve some of the burden placed on family members of the severely mentally ill. As Torrey (1997:77) notes, "One of the most difficult experiences for families with a mentally ill member is watching the person deteriorate psychiatrically without being able to do anything about it because of stringent involuntary commitment laws." Not only can hospital diversion programs take the place of hospitalization, in many cases they can better equip the family in their effort to care for ill relatives. Still, it becomes evident when comparing the NIMH statement with Lamb's that treating mentally ill individuals in the community is beneficial only if the proper supports are in place.

The literature on the topic of community versus institutional care is exhaustive. Many writers have addressed and various studies have targeted the pros and cons of each treatment method (Ruggeri et al., 2006; Ligon & Thyer, 2000; Granello, Granello, & Lee, 1999; Torrey, 1997; Warner, 1995). There appears to be a consensus that it is typically more beneficial and less detrimental for an individual experiencing acute mental illness to receive community-based care. This is the case only when the treatment in the community is appropriate and accessible. When describing the basic needs of people in the community with severe mental illness, Lamb (2001:7) claims, "Adequate, comprehensive, and accessible psychiatric and rehabilitative services need to be available and, when necessary, provided through outreach programs." The literature indicates that, for several reasons, our nation's cities and communities must provide adequate treatment for mentally ill citizens both in hospitals and in the community.

TYPES OF HOSPITAL DIVERSION PROGRAMS

A variety of hospital diversion programs are currently operating, and each has its strengths and limitations. All share the same goal of helping people thrive in the community and avoid institutionalization. Four of the most popular and well-researched programs are described in this section.

Assertive Community Treatment

One of the most popular community-based models for hospital diversion is the program for assertive community treatment (PACT), also called assertive community treatment (ACT) teams. Stein and Santos (1998:2) claim, "ACT is best conceptualized as a service delivery vehicle or system designed to furnish the latest, most effective and efficient treatments, rehabilitation, and support services conveniently as an integrated package." Much of the work performed by ACT/PACT staff involves case management and other supportive activities. This includes, among many other things, advocacy, completing applications for financial assistance, providing transportation to medical appointments, calling in and picking up prescriptions, and teaching daily living skills. However, there is still a large opportunity for interactions that are more clinical in nature because of the severity of illness, comorbid substance use and personality disturbance, and occurrence of daily life stressors that are common among ACT clients. One of the most significant ways in which ACT differs from traditional case management is that ACT staff directly provide treatment and rehabilitation.

ACT/PACT programs consist of multidisciplinary teams that provide services to individuals with severe mental illness who have not responded well to other forms of treatment, often because of noncompliance or difficulty accessing services. Typical ACT clients have primary mental health diagnoses on the schizophrenia or mood disorder spectrum. It is also common for them to have other comorbid conditions, such as substance abuse issues (Bond et al., 2001). Their mental illness and other characteristics, such as low income, limited support, unemployment, poor housing, and lack of transportation significantly reduce accessibility to needed mental health treatment. Thus a system of care that is mobile and comprehensive (i.e., similar to a psychiatric hospital) is indicated. A complete ACT team usually consists of a psychiatrist, psychologist, or clinical social worker; vocational rehabilitation specialist; substance abuse counselor; nurse; peer support specialists; and administrative assistants. These teams proactively meet with their clients in the community and provide a number of services.

Assertive community treatment is not just a philosophy or specific staff structure; it also consists of a particular protocol for service delivery that has been shown to be effective (Bond et al., 2001). The key components include multidisciplinary staffing, integration of services, a team approach, low patient-staff ratios, community contacts, medication management, focus on everyday problems in living, rapid access to client emergencies, assertive outreach, individualized services, and time-unlimited services (Bond et al., 2001). ACT also promotes recovery through community integration, vocational assistance, restoring family relationships, and providing opportunities for clients to lead groups and become peer support specialists.

Leonard Stein, Mary Ann Test, and their colleagues developed this model of treatment approximately thirty years ago in Madison, Wisconsin (Stein & Test, 1980). Since then ACT teams have been established across the globe (Bond et al., 2001). Various adaptations have been made to the original model in places with a geographic and demographic profile that differs from that of Madison.

Mobile Crisis Home Treatment

Mobile crisis home treatment (MCHT) teams, also called mobile crisis units or emergency services programs, generally provide services that are more focused on crisis assessment and referral to hospitals or other treatment settings. Their services are time limited, but just like an ACT program, services are provided twenty-four hours a day, and most of the interventions occur in the client's home. MCHT is most helpful for clients who are typically noncompliant with treatment recommendations and do not necessarily need to leave their home to become stable (i.e., their home environment is not the primary cause of or a significant contributor to their instability) (Heath, 2005). These teams help to reduce unnecessary arrests or medical attention (such as costly emergency room visits) by closely coordinating their services with police and emergency medical workers (Scott, 2000).

One of the disadvantages of MCHT and ACT programs is that they typically do not provide the needed structure and activity scheduling that severely mentally ill clients often need (Heath, 2005). They are also limited by their inability to provide interpersonal support, although some ACT programs offer group therapy and social outings. Even so, clients often prefer these programs because they are the least restrictive and most convenient.

Partial Hospitalization

Partial hospitalization and psychosocial rehabilitation programs attempt to provide the structure, activity, interpersonal contact, and monitoring that clients typically receive in an inpatient setting. These programs are helpful in that they can provide respite from a stressful home environment for the client and a break for family members who are caring for the individual (Heath, 2005). They also offer group therapy, job training, education, and opportunities for community integration.

Unfortunately many individuals who are experiencing acute symptomatology may be disruptive during the daily activities or not be able to tolerate the amount of activity and interpersonal contact that occurs during the four to five hours of the program. Furthermore these programs provide little benefit to clients who have difficulty communicating with others or do not have the insight necessary to participate in either process or education groups. Another aspect of these programs is that clients can drop out or be discharged owing to poor attendance, behavior problems, or the inability to demonstrate that they are benefiting. Typically a good screening process prior to admission to the program will prevent some of these incidences, but in the cases where an individual is discharged he or she may lose the important monitoring aspect of the program and be permitted to decompensate further and without notice.

Crisis Stabilization

Crisis stabilization programs typically come in two forms: home based and center based. Center-based programs offer twenty-four-hour monitoring of individuals who are experiencing acute psychiatric disturbance, require substance detoxification, or pose a mild to moderate suicide or homicide risk. These individuals typically do not meet criteria for hospitalization because they have not been shown to be an imminent danger to themselves or others, but they will require inpatient care if the stabilization program is not successful. These programs are also used as a step-down program from inpatient treatment.

Home-based crisis stabilization programs are similar to ACT and MCHT programs in that they provide interventions in the client's home and assist clients with getting to their medical and psychiatric appointments or other services that will facilitate their stabilization. Typically the programs are staffed by individuals with bachelor's or master's degrees in mental health or social work. Some programs have an integrated treatment team comprising nurses, psychologists, social workers, counselors, or rehabilitation workers. Staff members assess the referred individual's crisis situation and determine the person's appropriateness for crisis stabilization. If the individual does not yet meet criteria for inpatient care and does not require twenty-four-hour monitoring but needs a level of care that is more intensive than other programs (e.g., ACT or intensive case management), he or she will be admitted. This may also be an option for the individual who cannot participate in partial hospitalization.

Each hospital diversion program has a unique role in the mental health care system, and each is necessary for continuity of care. The common denominator is that ACT, MCHT, partial hospitalization, and crisis stabilization staff are frequently confronted with unstable or decompensating clients who need a higher level of clinical assistance until they are restored to their normal level of functioning. Fortunately studies targeting the effectiveness of these programs are beginning to emerge.

DO HOSPITAL DIVERSION PROGRAMS WORK?

In general there is evidence that community-based treatment might be more desired and more effective than hospital-based care for some clients. Findings from one study suggest that users of a service with a well-developed community-oriented approach and with crisis intervention outside the hospital setting are more satisfied with the emergency interventions than are users of a mental health service relying mostly on hospital facilities during emergencies (Ruggeri et al., 2006). Another study compared early intervention by community services and standard hospital treatment. One hundred patients ages 16 to 65 years who were experiencing a psychiatric emergency were treated by either a multidisciplinary community-based team ($n = 48$) or conventional hospital-based psychiatric services (n = 52) and assessed over a three-month period. Patients referred to the community-based service showed greater improvement in symptoms and were more satisfied with services than were those in the hospital-based service. In fact, patients treated in the hospital spent eight times as many days as psychiatric inpatients as those treated in the community-based service (Merson et al., 1992).

The only hospital diversion program that has received significant attention in the literature is assertive community treatment. Partial hospitalization programs have been around for a few decades, but very few studies have looked at these programs. Likewise, crisis stabilization programs have received very little attention. The likely explanation is that crisis stabilization programs are relatively new, and the number of partial hospitalization and crisis stabilization programs has not been large enough to warrant empirical investigation.

Several studies have demonstrated the efficacy of the assertive community treatment model as an intervention for the severely mentally ill. Specifically it has been found to reduce the frequency of hospitalization (Bonsack et al., 2005; Ben-Porath, Peterson, & Piskur, 2004; Blow et al., 2000; Chinman et al., 1999; Tibbo, Chue, & Wright, 1999; Essock, Frisman, & Kontos, 1998; Stein & Test, 1980), improve quality of life (Chinman et al., 1999), decrease homelessness (McBride et al., 1998), and lower overall mental health care costs (Latimer 2011, 2005, 1999; Essock, Frisman, & Kontos, 1998). Crisis stabilization programs have also effectively reduced hospitalization (Reding & Raphelson, 1995; Zealberg, Santos, & Fisher, 1993), and partial hospitalization programs have been found to be effective in reducing hospitalization and decreasing symptom severity among individuals with severe mental illness (Husted & Wentler, 2000; Granello, Granello, & Lee, 1999).

There have been mixed results regarding assertive community treatment's ability to reduce symptomatology for severely mentally ill individuals. Jerrell (1999) reported that psychiatric symptoms were substantially reduced after six and eighteen months of ACT intervention in a sample of 122 individuals primarily diagnosed with schizophrenia or schizoaffective disorder. Stein & Test (1980) found similar results using a comparable sample. On the other hand, Drake and colleagues (1998) studied the effect of assertive community treatment versus standard case management services on several outcome variables over a three-year period with a sample of 223 dual-disordered individuals. The authors claimed there were no differences in the reduction of psychiatric symptoms or remission of substance use disorders. Also, Links and colleagues (2005) explored the reasons for ACT's apparent ineffectiveness in reducing the risk of suicide and suicidal behavior. Their results suggest that the traditional assertive community treatment strategies for targeting crisis prevention, such as checking for suicidal ideation regularly or intensive follow-up and monitoring, are not as effective for preventing suicide as interventions that target the ongoing vulnerabilities such as impulsivity, agitation, and hopelessness.

A meta-analysis of assertive community treatment revealed more conflicting results. For instance, Bond and colleagues (2001) summarized the findings of twenty-five randomized controlled trials looking at ACT program effectiveness. They reported that psychiatric hospital use decreased among ACT clients, compared to a control group, in seventeen studies while six studies showed no difference. The presence of symptoms was reduced in seven studies, but nine studies showed no difference. Furthermore, substance use decreased in two studies, but ACT was similar to control groups in its ability to reduce this behavior in four studies.

Although several factors could contribute to the less than perfect record of ACT program effectiveness in preventing hospitalization, improving symptom management, and decreasing substance use, one of the problems might be the absence of a strong clinical component in some programs. After witnessing the deterioration of the home-based program he developed and ran for years, a former executive director stated, "It is quite clear that alternatives to acute psychiatric hospitalization cannot survive without continued commitment to the concept by the leadership of the mental health structure in which they operate and both commitment and skill on the part of the clinical staff" (Polak, Kirby, & Deitchman, 1995:223).

Chinman and colleagues (1999) provide support for the idea that attention to clinical needs might be lacking in hospital diversion programs such as assertive community treatment. These researchers interviewed ACT clinicians and reported that the

> ACT clinicians either did not mention how they addressed their clients' psychotic symptoms or they stated that they brought their clients to the psychiatrist whenever a client was becoming more symptomatic. Perhaps ACT

clinicians are not familiar with ways to address psychotic symptoms beyond medication or are not comfortable talking to clients about their symptoms. This situation provides another opportunity for staff development. For example, cognitive-behavioral treatment has been extended to the treatment of psychosis and ACT clinicians may benefit from being trained in and using these methods with their clients. (157)

Many ACT teams, and other hospital diversion or acute care programs, might be negating the clinical aspects of treatment because they do not have appropriate staff, do not have adequate training, or are consumed with case management tasks.

In a study that measured the effectiveness of an assertive community treatment program over a period of three years, Ben-Porath, Peterson, and Piskur (2004) found that the program was highly effective for the first two years but became less effective between the second and third year. Specifically there was a significant decrease in inpatient bed days and emergency outpatient contacts between the year prior to ACT services and the first and second years of services, but there was an increase in the use of these extra services between the second and third years. Other studies have demonstrated poor long-term efficacy (Audini et al., 1994; Mulder, 1982), each of which suggests the most significant treatment gains occur in the first two years. This finding may indicate that the clients become somewhat stabilized as they secure housing and begin attending psychiatric appointments, but they eventually decompensate because their mental health issues have not received the same level of attention as housing, finances, and other concerns received.

One might ask why they do not just refer those who need psychotherapy or counseling to outpatient services. One problem is that ACT is considered a bundled service in most areas; this means the insurance provider (usually Medicaid) will not pay for any other mental health service because it is presumed that the ACT/PACT team will provide all services (Human Services, 2008). For this reason and others, it is important that ACT programs provide more psychological services, such as suicide/homicide assessment, brief and long-term therapy, and crisis intervention. This might require the inclusion of more psychologists, psychiatric nurses, or clinical social workers in the formation of ACT teams. In cases where these persons are already employed, it is important that they continue to use their clinical skills and abstain from focusing entirely on administrative or case management tasks, which often happens as these persons are often the program coordinators. Another option is to equip each team member, no matter what discipline he or she may represent, with basic and effective therapeutic tools for facilitating crisis intervention and for combating decompensation with severely mentally ill clients.

2

Integrative and Multimodal Treatment

WHEN PROVIDING MENTAL HEALTH TREATMENT, it is typically important to have an underlying theoretical framework that will guide the various interventions in a purposeful manner. For instance, a cognitive therapist will set out to understand more clearly the underlying thoughts or assumptions that drive an individual's behavior and eventually assist the person in challenging any assumptions that are faulty. The cognitive therapist will view most problems through this thought-behavior-consequence lens. Likewise, therapists who maintain other theoretical orientations have likely become comfortable with a particular perspective and approach clinical issues accordingly.

There is nothing wrong with limiting oneself to one theoretical or treatment model (e.g., cognitive, interpersonal, systems, dynamic); in fact this may be necessary to achieve expertise in the use of a particular theory or set of techniques. However, it can be difficult to accurately conceptualize the incredible sum of diverse human behaviors with one perspective. Brendel (2003:565) expresses this idea as follows: "Human action and experience usually are far too complex to be captured adequately in explanations which appeal only to the concepts and tools of a single scientific discipline." Human behavior is determined by multiple factors, and it is often necessary to consider more than one perspective to form an accurate assessment and establish a successful treatment plan.

Concentrating on one framework or set of treatment strategies may result in the exclusion of helpful strategies that belong to other conceptual models. For instance, a strict cognitive or behavior perspective might negate important issues within the client's system (family, work, peers) and a strict solution-focused approach might negate important underlying processes such as maladaptive schemas or unconscious conflicts or motivations. Fosha (2004:68) explains, "People are messy and multimodal, complex and chaotic systems. Thus, change as an organic process is invariably complex and multifaceted." The complicated issues that individuals experiencing severe mental illness often present with are seldom explainable or treatable through a unimodal or a nonintegrated framework.

INTEGRATIVE TREATMENT

Over the past decade there has been an increasingly popular shift away from the dogmatic adherence to one therapy orientation toward models of integration (Goldfried, Pachankis, & Bell, 2005). In 2009 Barlow suggested that "the age of schools of psychotherapy has been over for about five years." Much has been written about this topic beginning at least as early as the 1960s, leading to the founding of the Society for the Exploration of Psychotherapy Integration in 1983. This society created the *Journal of Psychotherapy Integration* and held annual international meetings (Lazarus, 2005a). In the late 1990s therapists and authors such as John Preston (2006) began describing ways to combine cognitive, humanistic, psychodynamic, neurobehavioral, and other approaches to meet the demands of managed care and the needs of clients.

Anchin (2008:19) describes psychotherapy integration as a "scientific paradigm." It is a movement that is pervasive and likely to continue to gain momentum. According to Norcross, Hedges, and Castle (2002), approximately 36 percent of clinical psychologists claimed to have an eclectic or integrative orientation in 2001. Multiple integrative psychotherapy models currently exist, and therapists are continually publishing new, creative combinations of treatment strategies.

Psychotherapy integration comes in many forms. In general the approaches fall into three categories: assimilative integration, sequential and parallel integration, and eclecticism. In assimilative integration the therapist espouses a primary theoretical orientation and selectively integrates perspectives or techniques from one or more different theoretical orientations (Messer, 1992). Sequential integration involves combining two or more treatment models in distinct phases. Each phase consists of a pure treatment model that has been chosen to meet the individual's needs (Schottenbauer, Glass, & Arnkoff, 2005).

Eclecticism is atheoretical and therefore lacks a conceptual framework to guide the use of particular interventions. However, according to Lampropoulos (2000), eclectic psychotherapy must include important common factors (i.e., therapeutic alliance, supportive environment, empathy, exploration, insight, catharsis, and problem confrontation). He suggests that these essential therapeutic change agents can guide eclectic treatment, which may otherwise be conducted in a less than meaningful way.

Psychopathology-matched eclecticism represents the empirically supported treatment movement and involves the selection of specific strategies that have been found effective for particular problems (Lampropoulos, 2000). Personality-matched eclecticism also focuses on matching effective treatments with appropriate candidates. Support for this approach comes from the work of Beutler and his colleagues (Beutler et al., 1999; Fisher, Beutler, & Williams, 1999; Beutler & Clarkin, 1990; Beutler, 1983), who developed an eclectic treatment model called systematic treatment selection (STS). Their integrative work stems from the belief that the predominant way of approaching psychotherapy is flawed because of an unsupported focus on manualized treatment based on one conceptual model and a lack of attention to the universal factors of change. They explain:

> These collective failures of research, theory, and practice suggest a need for integrative approaches wherein specific interventions can be designed for specific purposes, patients, populations, and conditions. A useful integrative approach, however, must account for the universe of factors that contribute to psychotherapeutic change rather than focusing on the limited variables associated with a single theoretical model. (Beutler, Consoli, & Lane, 2005:122)

The STS model, which has received empirical support (Beutler et al., 2003; Beutler, Clarkin, & Bongar, 2000; Beutler & Harwood, 2000), developed through a series of studies (Beutler, Clarkin, & Bongar, 2000; Beutler, Mohr, et al., 1991; Beutler, Engle, et al., 1991; Calvert, Beutler, & Crago, 1988; Beutler & Mitchell, 1981). It describes several characteristic domains with which to match appropriate treatments with particular clients.

Integrative treatments are used to address several different diagnoses. For instance, a sequential integration approach that combined cognitive-behavioral and psychodynamic-interpersonal treatment (one treatment before the other) produced substantial short- and long term gains in a group of individuals with anxiety or depression (Shapiro & Firth, 1987; Shapiro & Firth-Cozens, 1990). Another integrative treatment that targeted generalized anxiety disorder with cognitive-behavioral therapy (CBT) and interpersonal/emotional processing therapy was found to be effective (Newman, Castonguay, & Borkovec, 2002). Additionally, dialectical behavior therapy (DBT), which includes cognitive-behavioral, mindfulness, and dialectic components, has received support as an effective treatment for many conditions (borderline personality, alcohol dependence, eating disorders, and depression) in several settings (inpatient hospital, forensic hospital, Veterans Administration clinics, and outpatient) (Schottenbauer, Glass, & Arnkoff, 2005).

The efficacy of several other integrative psychotherapy approaches that address specific clinical populations and presenting problems has been documented (Schottenbauer, Glass, & Arnkoff, 2005). For instance, Gersons and colleagues (2000) and Lindauer and colleagues (2005) have demonstrated the efficacy of a treatment method for posttraumatic stress disorder (PTSD) called brief eclectic psychotherapy (BEP) that combines cognitive-behavioral and psychodynamic strategies. BEP includes five essential elements: psychoeducation, imaginary guidance, writing assignments, meaning making, and a farewell letter. Process-experiential therapy integrates process-directive, experiential, and client-centered interventions. Similarly, functional analytic psychotherapy is a form of cognitive therapy that is supplemented by ongoing behavior analysis of the therapeutic relationship between the client and the treatment provider. Both treatments have been found to be more effective than nonintegrated approaches in reducing symptoms of depression (Goldman, Greenberg, and Angus, 2006; Kohlenberg et al., 2002). Another integrative treatment, mindfulness-based cognitive therapy for depression, which emphasizes awareness of thoughts and feelings, reduced relapse of depressive symptoms in a group of clients who have had more than three depressive episodes (Ma & Teasdale, 2004; Teasdale et al., 2000). McMinn & Campbell (2007) have developed an integrative psychotherapy approach that begins with behavioral interventions and moves from cognitive interventions to schema-focused and relationship-focused interventions. Other integrative therapies include Magnavita and Carlson's (2003) short-term restructuring psychotherapy; McCullough's

(2003) cognitive-behavioral analysis system of psychotherapy for chronic depression; Linehan's (1993b) dialectical behavior therapy; Anchin's (2003) cybernetic systems, existential-phenomenology, and solution-focused narrative; and Levenson's (2003) time-limited dynamic psychotherapy. Altogether at least thirty different psychotherapy integration models have been studied, and several others are in the process of receiving empirical support (Schottenbauer, Glass, & Arnkoff, 2005).

MULTIMODAL THERAPY

Arnold Lazarus developed multimodal therapy (1981, 1986, 1989, 1997, 2000), which is a psychotherapy approach based on the same underlying principles of integration described above and promises to be both brief and comprehensive. Multimodal therapy (MMT) is considered a form of technical eclecticism because treatment components from various theoretical models, especially cognitive-behavioral, are prescribed as long as they are not conflicting (Lazarus, 2005a). Lazarus uses the techniques found in various approaches to target the multiple dimensions of a client's existence. In explaining the development of the model, Lazarus (2005a:106) writes:

> Emphasis was placed on the fact that, at a base, we are biological organisms (neurophysiological/biochemical entities) who behave (act and react), emote (experience affective responses), sense (respond to tactile, olfactory, gustatory, visual, and auditory stimuli), imagine (conjure up sights, sounds, and other events in our mind's eye), think (entertain beliefs, opinions, values, and attitudes), and interact with one another (enjoy, tolerate, or suffer various interpersonal relationships).

Lazarus conceptualizes the complexity of human beings and recognizes the need to account for the multiple variables that clients bring to the psychotherapy encounter. Others have echoed this perspective. For instance, Preston (2006) suggests there are a number of "psychological liabilities" that may cause an individual to have difficulty coping with stress. These are significant privation (homelessness, malnourishment, poverty), lack of appropriate social supports, lack of adequate social skills (communication, problem solving), factors that interfere with emotional healing (negative schemas, emotional instability, overdefensiveness), and neurobiological factors. O'Connor (2003) provides a similar list of vulnerabilities that make individuals susceptible to depression: early loss or trauma, unstable self-esteem, pessimistic thinking, poor interpersonal skills, and lack of social supports.

Multimodal therapists not only try to determine the modalities in which the client is having difficulty but also evaluate which ones the client is willing to work on and join them at this place. The therapist moves from modality to modality, as the client permits, until each area of concern is addressed. Even though several aspects of the client receive attention, the majority of the interventions are cognitive-behavioral in nature. As Lazarus (2005a:113) notes, "In a sense, the term 'multimodal therapy' is a misnomer because while the assessment is multimodal, the treatment is cognitive-behavioral and draws, whenever possible, on empirically supported methods." It is the emphasis on ensuring that each aspect, or modality, of the client is assessed and no important issue is left untreated that makes multimodal therapy a unique choice for clinicians.

One of the basic premises of the multimodal approach is that it is not necessary to fully comprehend why someone is having difficulties to be of help to them. According to Lazarus (1997:38), "Issues pertaining to etiology and causality are poorly understood. Moreover, we do not require a precise explanation of what caused a problem in order to remedy it." Much time can be wasted in the pursuit of the best explanatory model for an individual's symptoms, and this simply prolongs their plight. In brief therapy settings, such as crisis intervention, no time can be wasted; therefore when assessing the areas in which there are difficulties, there is no need to take a journey into the past to determine how the various problems developed. The truth is that mental health professionals are only making educated guesses, and it is impossible to capture the whole story given the complexity of the human experience.

Lazarus (1997) uses the acronym BASIC I.D. to help clinicians remember the seven modalities of an individual's life that should be assessed and ultimately addressed through multimodal therapy. BASIC I.D. stands for the behavior, affect, sensation and imagery experiences, cognition, interpersonal experiences, and drugs/biology within a particular person. With the behavior modality, clinicians are interested in client behaviors or actions that are causing problems. At times actions need to be increased or decreased, done more effectively, or eliminated. Often new actions need to be introduced as an alternative to maladaptive ones. For instance, use of a substance as a means to cope with stress might be replaced with deep breathing, exercise, or meditation.

The affect modality refers to the multiple emotions that a person experiences, including anger, sadness, fear, joy, and so on. The clinician is tasked with assessing the individual's prominent emotional states and linking these to the thoughts and behaviors associated with them. For instance, a person who presents as severely depressed might frequently experience feelings of sadness and loneliness. This might be triggered by recurring thoughts and images of a loved one who recently passed away, and it might result in the person becoming withdrawn, crying excessively, or even threatening to take a lethal dose of a prescribed medication.

Lazarus introduces two less commonly targeted modalities into the treatment picture by emphasizing sensation and imagery. Sensation includes physical experiences such as pain, tension, nausea, comfort, or level of energy. Imagery includes the pictures that enter the mind either randomly or during particular situations. These might come in the form of flashbacks, fantasies, or dreams. Issues related to imagery can be found in some anxiety disorders (e.g., PTSD) and other conditions. In many cases sensation and imagery can be used to target other modalities (e.g., cognitive or interpersonal) that might not be as accessible.

Cognition is a modality that clinicians frequently target. A person's thoughts, assumptions, and way of interpreting the events around them can have a significant influence on his or her emotional and social well-being. It is important for clinicians to assess the attitudes, beliefs, values, and thought process of the individual being treated so that dysfunctional or maladaptive thinking can be addressed. Sometimes this is the focus area used to challenge a psychotic process or cycle of depression. At other times this modality is accessed very early to improve an individual's motivation to engage in the treatment process.

The final two aspects of the individual that multimodal therapy targets are interpersonal or social health and biological health. Clinicians want to know the characteristics of the person's current and past relationships (abuse history, quality of social skills, ability to have needs met and meet needs of others) as well as thoughts and feelings about future relationships. It is also important to learn about the person's sense of social support and whether or not the person feels there are people who can be trusted and relied on.

In many cases the etiology of mental health issues is found in a person's biological makeup. Furthermore, an individual's physical health effects his or her psychological health, and vice versa. Physical health is affected by a person's behavior (sleep, exercise, hygiene) as well as the substances introduced into the person's body (medications, foods, drugs, environmental toxins). Physical health needs are typically addressed prior to mental health treatment, and they most certainly cannot be ignored.

According to Lazarus (1997), the formula for brief and comprehensive psychotherapy involves a four-step process. First, assess for problems in each of the seven modalities described above. Second, work with the client to choose three or four problems to target during therapy. Third, have the client address any physical health concerns and obtain medication as needed. And last, use empirically validated interventions to resolve specific problems (see Lazarus, 1997, for more about multimodal therapy).

Although this broadly scoped and personalized model of psychotherapy does not lend itself well to outcome studies, it has received empirical support. For instance, Kwee (1984) studied the implementation of multimodal treatment regimens with eighty-four hospitalized patients with obsessive-compulsive disorders and extensive phobias who were previously refractory to treatment in Holland. The multimodal treatment resulted in substantial short- and long-term gains. Kwee and Kwee-Taams (1994) produced even better results in an additional study. Freidmann and Silvers (1977) also reported positive and sustained results following multimodal treatment of a similar population. Further evidence of the effectiveness of multimodal therapy comes from a study of a successful multimodal exposure-based group treatment for veterans with PTSD in which there were improvements in a broad range of problem areas (Rademaker, Vermetten, & Kleber, 2009).

Other clinicians have effectively used a multimodal treatment approach. For example, O'Connor (2003) offers an integrative, multimodal approach to treating depression that involves facilitating healthy regulation of emotions, increasing awareness and understanding of emotions, teaching interpersonal skills, challenging depressive thinking, improving self-care, and offering antidepressant medication. He provides the following rationale for this approach: "Trying to understand depression exclusively from a single perspective—for instance, a cognitive-behavioral, psychodynamic, or biochemical point of view—necessarily limits our understanding and our ability to help our patients. Rather, we must be willing to take the best knowledge from many different points of view and shape it into practice guidelines" (131).

Likewise, Randal, Simpson, and Laidlaw (2003) demonstrate the efficacy of a recovery-focused treatment program targeting patients along the schizophrenia spectrum. This multimodal approach significantly reduced overall scores on the Positive and Negative Symptoms Scale (PANSS) and decreased deviant behavior in this sample. Additionally, Zuercher-White (1997) indicate there is consensus among a number of researchers that integrated, multimodal treatment of panic disorder is most effective. The necessary components include psychoeducation, breathing retraining, interoceptive exposure, in vivo exposure, cognitive restructuring, and relapse prevention.

In sum, the appeal of working within an integrative and multimodal framework is clear: the therapist feels better equipped to facilitate change. According to Brendel (2003:565), with the integrative approach, "The clinician has a broad and unrestricted set of tools with which to explain why people act as they do, and to integrate seemingly different tools in order to treat patients more sensitively and effectively." Another important aspect of the integrative treatment and the multimodal approach is a focus on outcome and the use of empirically supported treatment tools. Lazarus (2005b:151) states, "It seems that the current emphasis in enlightened circles has turned to empirically supported methods and the use of manuals in psychotherapy research and practice." Furthermore, as suggested by one group of integrationists, "When outcome-informed, a clinician is limited only by practical and ethical considerations and their creativity" (Miller, Duncan, & Hubble, 2005:90).

This brief review of integrative treatment in general and multimodal therapy more specifically is included to provide a context and rationale for the acute psychiatric care model described later in this book.

3

Severe Mental Illness Treatment Literature

AN OVERVIEW

MUCH EFFORT HAS GONE INTO developing an accurate and useful definition of severe mental illness. A National Institute of Mental Health working group used three criteria to define severe mental illness: a diagnosis of nonorganic psychosis or personality disorder; a long history of previous hospitalizations or outpatient treatment; and disability that includes dangerous or disturbing social behavior, moderate impairment in work and nonwork activities, and mild impairment in basic needs (NIMH, 1987). Some researchers (e.g., Parabiaghi et al., 2006; Ruggeri et al., 2000) have suggested a three-dimensional operational definition that includes psychiatric diagnosis, duration of service contact of two years or more, and Global Assessment of Functioning score of 50 or less. The majority of individuals who use hospital diversion programs meet these criteria. Individuals who utilize hospital diversion programs but are not considered severely mentally ill most likely experience chronic depression, anxiety, or substance abuse issues that cause frequent crises.

Individuals who are characterized as experiencing a serious mental illness make up a small proportion of the mentally ill population in general (Kessler et al., 2005). However, according to the National Institute of Mental Health (2008), the main burden of mental illness is concentrated in this group. This is one reason why it is essential to develop and disseminate effective treatments.

Much has been written about treating the severely mentally ill. Recently a shift has occurred in the language surrounding this population in both scholarly texts and clinical settings. There has been an increase in expressions of hope and optimism as mental health professionals adopt a philosophy of recovery. The severely mentally ill are no longer seen as people who simply need to be contained and secluded from society. More people are realizing that those with schizophrenia, bipolar disorder, and similar illnesses can be great contributors to their communities. Many already work and live normal, productive lives, but these individuals are not always acknowledged. Recovery goes beyond symptom management and includes reaching a new, higher level of functioning. Fortunately this is the focus of many treatment programs today.

Multidisciplinary treatment teams, access to crisis support, and therapeutic intervention that assists individuals in overcoming cognitive, behavioral, and interpersonal deficits are necessary components of effective intervention for this population. According to Mitchell (2004:281), "Treatment [for severe mental illness] should aim to restore the person to full health and a meaningful life. Prevention of suicide must be a central goal. Integration of a range of health professionals, as well as family and friends, is required." It can be a tall order to help restore a person with severe mental illness to a fully healthy and meaningful life; this could be why some continue to shy away from the recovery movement. This type of treatment requires a community that expresses hopefulness as well as a competent crew of service providers. In a study that assessed the necessary clinical competencies for effectively providing care to the severely mentally ill through community-based programs, professionals representing several disciplines developed a list of thirty-seven needed competencies. Some of the competencies listed are being skilled in using current psychosocial/psychiatric rehabilitation approaches; being able to teach illness self-management skills; and being able to evaluate client preferences regarding interventions that have been successful in the past. The researchers claim that clinicians providing care to this population do not currently demonstrate most competencies (Young et al., 2000).

Although the treatment process can be challenging at times, individuals with severe mental illness often respond favorably to therapy. Descriptions of several treatment approaches, including cognitive-behavioral therapy, dialectical-behavior therapy, multisystemic treatment, short-term dynamic psychotherapy, personal therapy, interpersonal therapy, and social skills training, can be found in Hofmann and Tompson's (2002) text, *Treating Chronic and Severe Mental Disorders: A Handbook of Empirically Supported Interventions*. Clearly there are several treatments that work.

A brief overview of the research addressing treatment of the various disorders often associated with severe mental illness is given below. Several modalities of empirically supported treatments are covered to illustrate the need for a multimodal approach to treating this clinical population. The evidence related to brief, crisis, or acute phase treatment is emphasized. This literature review is also intended to support Lazarus's claim that "there does not appear to be a single instance wherein a blend of different theories produced a more powerful technique, but there are numerous cases where techniques drawn from different disciplines have enriched clinicians' armamentaria" (1995:27). Examples of therapeutic strategies used to address common symptoms of various severe mental illnesses are discussed in the following sections. Most treatments are born out of a cognitive-behavioral or social learning theoretical framework.

SCHIZOPHRENIA AND SCHIZOAFFECTIVE DISORDER

Schizophrenia and schizoaffective disorder are typically combined in both outcome studies and theoretical and clinical discussions. By itself, schizoaffective disorder has received very little attention in the empirical literature while schizophrenia has been studied extensively for several years. One reason for this discrepancy could be the continued debate over whether schizoaffective disorder is a unique, legitimate condition different from schizophrenia or bipolar disorder (Whaley, 2002; Vogl & Zaudig, 1985; Himmelhoch et al., 1981; Pope et al., 1980). This review will discuss interventions for schizophrenia and schizoaffective disorder together to be consistent with the current literature.

While several antipsychotic medications have been proven as a valuable, if not essential, treatment for clients in the acute phase of schizophrenia, adjunctive treatment, particularly psychosocial interventions, is usually also required for faster and more complete stabilization (Zhao & Jin, 2010; Kane, 1997; Kane & McGlashan, 1995). Personal therapy (Hogarty, 2002), cognitive-behavioral family treatment (Falloon, 2002), social skills training (Pratt & Mueser, 2002), problem-solving training (Falloon et al., 2007), individual cognitive-behavioral therapy (Tarrier & Haddock, 2002), and integrative and multimodal treatment approaches (Tillman, 2008; Randal, Simpson, & Laidlaw, 2003) have received empirical support as psychological treatments for schizophrenia. While social skills training, problem-solving training, and personal therapy improve overall functioning and prevent relapse during the nonacute period of the illness, individual and family-oriented cognitive-behavioral treatments have demonstrated success in improving positive and negative symptoms and expediting stability during both the acute and nonacute phases (Mastroeni et al., 2005; Lewis et al., 2002; Tarrier et al., 1993, 2000; Heinssen, Liberman, & Kopelowicz, 2000; Sensky et al., 2000; Haddock et al., 1999; Hogarty et al., 1986, 1991, 1997; Drury et al., 1996a, 1996b). Therefore, although often necessary, pharmacological intervention is not the only option clinicians can offer an individual with schizophrenia experiencing acute symptomatology.

One approach that can be highly beneficial is cognitive-behavioral therapy. CBT has a reputation in the fields of psychology and counseling as an effective treatment for mood and anxiety disorders, but the notion that it can be used to address more complicated symptoms such as delusions and hallucinations may not be as popular. Several books and articles discuss CBT for psychotic disorders (e.g., Kingdon & Turkington, 2005; Tarrier & Haddock, 2002; Grech, 2002; Baker, 2000), and there is empirical support for this approach to treating psychosis (Bechdolf et al., 2005; Tarrier et al., 1998). The most frequently used cognitive-behavioral interventions for schizophrenia patients include development of a collaborative understanding of the nature of the illness, identification of factors exacerbating symptoms, learning and strengthening skills for coping with and reducing symptoms and stress, reducing physiological arousal, testing key beliefs that may be supporting delusional thinking, and development of problem-solving strategies to reduce relapse (Psychosocial interventions, 2005). Tarrier & Haddock (2002:81–86) provide a detailed description of a cognitive-behavioral treatment of schizophrenia that consists of four main focus areas and several related strategies: coping enhancement and compensation strategies (attention switching and narrowing, increased activity levels, social engagement and disengagement, modified self statements, and internal dialogue); dearousing techniques (breathing retraining, relaxation strategies, self-soothing); increasing reality or source monitoring (awareness training, focusing, and self-monitoring); belief and attribution modification (examination of beliefs and reattribution, belief modification, reality testing, and behavioral experiments).

Researchers and clinicians have demonstrated success in treating acutely ill psychotic patients with cognitive therapy approaches. In one study, individuals in a CBT group experienced a significantly faster and more complete recovery from a psychotic episode compared to those in the control group, who received a structured activities program and nonspecific counseling. The treatment group received intensive CBT, which consisted of individual, group, and family sessions as well as a structured activities program. The therapy specifically targeted the modification of delusional beliefs and associated distress, negative symptoms, and relapse prevention (Drury et al., 1996a, 1996b). A treatment called cognitive analytic therapy (CAT) was found to be effective in reducing "disturbed and non-compliant behavior" with some patients with "post-acute manic psychosis" (Kerr, 2001). Cognitive enhancement therapy (CET), which combines supportive therapy with social skills and cognitive remediation training, has also shown promise as an effective treatment for individuals with schizophrenia (Miller & Mason, 2004).

It has been suggested that a parallel process of working with patients and working with families will be most effective during the acute stage of psychotic illness (Grawe et al., 2006; Miller & Mason, 1999). According to Falloon and colleagues (1999), adding psychosocial family interventions to pharmacotherapy and case management results in multiple positive outcomes for those with psychotic disorders including clinical, social, family and economic benefits. Falloon (2002) describes an intervention that focuses on educating the family of the schizophrenic client. The primary goals of cognitive-behavioral family therapy are to decrease the overall stress and improve the problem-solving capacity of the family unit. Various strategies are used, including education about the illness, communication training, problem-solving training, teaching of cognitive-behavioral strategies (e.g., relaxation training, cognitive restructuring, anger management), social skills training, and crisis intervention. Also an effort is made to employ the client's family and other supports as a team of cotherapists who reinforce the various skills being taught by the clinician. The overall health of the family unit is emphasized because it is believed that as the family becomes more adept at handling stress and resolving problems, the client will be less vulnerable to relapse.

More evidence by Doane and colleagues (1986) suggests it is important to include family members in the treatment of schizophrenia. These researchers studied the effects of individual versus family treatment in a sample of thirty-three people diagnosed with schizophrenia. After three months the number of critical statements and noncritical, intrusive remarks significantly decreased for parents in the family treatment group. An increase in the number of critical and/or intrusive remarks for parents in the individual treatment group was associated with an increased risk for relapse. According to the researchers, these results suggest that a behaviorally oriented, problem-solving family approach that teaches families concrete ways of solving problems and reduces the amount of negative emotional relating between family members may reduce relapse.

Several other conditions or problematic behaviors often coexist with psychotic disorders. According to Huguelet, Mohr, and Borras (2009:307), "Schizophrenia and other psychoses affect the whole life of patients [and] consequently, treatments should comprehensively cover all affected fields." One of the common comorbid issues is substance abuse; thus treatment that targets addictive behavior and related social concerns is often necessary. The benefits of adding an integrated psychological and psychosocial treatment program to routine psychiatric care for patients with schizophrenia and substance use disorders has been demonstrated (Barrowclough et al., 2001). Barrowclough and colleagues compared routine care with an intervention that involved motivational interviewing and integrated individual and family-oriented cognitive therapy in a sample of fifteen patients. The integrated treatment program resulted in significantly greater improvement in patients' general functioning compared to routine care alone at the end of treatment and twelve months after the beginning of the study. The program reduced positive symptoms and symptom exacerbations and increased the percent of days of abstinence from drugs or alcohol over the twelve-month period from baseline to follow-up. An eighteen-month follow-up revealed that the treatment program was superior to routine care on outcomes related to illness and service use (Haddock et al., 2003).

Many other researchers and clinicians have recognized the need to target multiple areas of an individual's life. For instance, Tillman (2008) has proposed another integrative approach. This author suggests that information gleaned from an internationally recognized intensive, psychodynamically oriented treatment center called Austen Riggs indicates the need for a model that combines individual psychodynamic psychotherapy, psychopharmacology, family systems approaches, and intensive psychosocial engagement. While the benefits of medication, family therapy, and psychosocial treatment are well documented, the efficacy of psychodynamic treatment has been questioned (Fenton, 2000; Eells, 2000). Another example of integration involves a comprehensive, community-based treatment program for patients with schizophrenia and schizoaffective disorders titled "Integrated Care," which significantly improved social functioning and patient satisfaction with treatment (Malm et al., 2003). Shared decision making and patient empowerment were emphasized in this assertive community treatment program that combined antipsychotic medication, family interventions, and social skills training.

Further evidence for the efficacy of integrating treatment strategies comes from Randal, Simpson, and Laidlaw (2003), who demonstrate the ability of a recovery-focused multimodal treatment program to significantly reduce overall scores on the Positive and Negative Symptoms Scale as well as decrease deviant behavior in a sample of patients diagnosed with schizophrenia or schizoaffective disorder. The treatment consisted of psychoeducational, cognitive-behavioral, interpersonal, supportive, and spiritual components implemented under an overarching recovery framework. Specific focuses included the development of a strong therapeutic alliance, increased hopefulness and motivation, affect regulation, reality testing or challenging thought distortion, restoring spirituality, and improving interpersonal skills.

It is important to note that individuals who experience psychotic symptoms are at a higher risk than the general population for self-harm. Bechdolf and colleagues (2003) investigated the determinants of subjective quality of life among patients with schizophrenia. They concluded that treatments that facilitate improvements in depressive symptoms, negative coping style, social support, and self-efficacy may be most effective in improving quality of life. These data correspond well with a study that examined the correlates of self-harm behavior among acutely ill patients with schizophrenia. In this study patients with a history of self-harm had significantly greater symptoms of depression, greater suicidal thoughts, increased numbers of hospital admissions, and greater duration of illness compared to patients without a history of self-harm (Simms et al., 2007).

Finally, engagement in the treatment process can be challenging with psychotic individuals. Fortunately, motivational interviewing (MI) strate-gies, such as those described by Miller and Rollnick (2002), can be used in the treatment of individuals with schizophrenia or schizoaffective disorder. McCracken & Corrigan (2008) have suggested guidelines for using an MI approach to improve medication adherence with this clinical population. The primary goals are to engage the individual through expressing empa-thy and communicating acceptance, help the client identify goals, and con-duct a cost-benefit discussion of how taking medication might help them achieve their goals. These authors state that the entire treatment team (psy-chiatrist, counselor, case manager, etc.) should use MI principles and activi-ties regularly in their effort to encourage medication adherence.

BIPOLAR AND MAJOR DEPRESSIVE DISORDER

Bipolar disorder and major depression are the two disorders most highly as-sociated with risk for completed suicide (Brown et al., 2000). Therefore it is imperative that people with these illnesses learn symptom-management skills to prevent decompensation, and that solid clinical care is provided in times of crisis. Several pharmacological and psychosocial interventions have shown promise in treating various aspects of these conditions, and a combination of the two is most commonly seen. However, much is yet to be determined regarding the etiology and treatment of mood disorders.

Bipolar disorder is among the mental health conditions with the most substantial amount of evidence suggesting a biological etiology (Craddock & Forty, 2006). Naturally the primary treatment for this condition, espe-cially the manic phase, is medication. The question of which drugs are most efficacious in controlling symptoms in both the manic and depressed phases of the illness has been heavily researched (Sachs & Gardner-Schuster, 2007; Krüger, Young, & Bräunig, 2005; Post et al., 2003; Goldberg & Truman, 2003; Baldessarini et al., 2002). Lithium, valproate, and several atypical an-tipsychotics continue to be recommended as first-line treatments for acute mania, while quetiapine monotherapy is currently recommended as the first-line pharmacological treatment of bipolar depression (Yatham et al., 2006). In spite of the emphasis on somatic treatment options, other therapies, such as cognitive-behavioral, psychoeducational, interpersonal, and family therapy, have also been proven effective in the treatment of bipolar disorder (Colom & Vieta, 2004; Huxley, Parikh, & Baldessarini, 2000).

According to Mitchell (2004:281), "The varied nature of BD [or bipolar disorder] requires a broad range of interventions." Among these is psychotherapy. While psychoactive medication remains the primary intervention for symptom management, psychological interventions typically address both the reduction of symptoms and functional recovery (Colom & Vieta, 2004). Poor social functioning, especially job functioning, predicted a shorter period of time before symptom relapse among bipolar patients in one study (Gitlin et al., 1995). Medication nonadherence has also been identified as a major factor in the occurrence of symptom relapse (Keck et al., 1998; Miklowitz et al., 1988). Therefore, as Miklowitz (2001) suggests, the primary role of psychotherapy in the treatment of bipolar disorder is to teach symptom-management skills, augment social and occupational role functioning, and keep patients adherent to their medication regimens.

The Royal Australian and New Zealand College of Psychiatrists clinical practice guidelines team reviewed the treatment outcome literature, consulted with practitioners and consumers, and recommended the following strategies as evidenced-based practice for treating bipolar disorder (Mitchell, 2004). For the acute mania stage of the illness, pharmacological treatment (e.g., lithium, carbamazepine, valproate) is recommended as the primary mode of intervention. When the patient presents in the acutely depressed phase of the illness, a combination of drug treatment (e.g., lamotrigine, selective serotonin reuptake inhibitors [SSRIs], antipsychotics for psychotic bipolar depression) and psychological treatments (e.g., psychoeducation, cognitive therapy, schema therapy, interpersonal and social rhythm therapy, group therapy, or family-focused treatment) should be used. Mitchell notes that the psychological treatments "may be applied in combination in clinical practice" (290).

In accordance with the guidelines described above, most studies have assessed the effects of combination therapies for bipolar disorder. The combination of drug therapy and cognitive therapy was found to more effectively decrease the recurrence of symptom episodes, improve affective stability, and improve medication adherence than routine care with medication among one sample of bipolar patients (Lam et al., 2000). As with schizophrenia, bipolar treatment programs typically attend to the issue of treatment adherence. In a study by Cochran (1984), cognitive therapy that focused on restructuring cognitions related to medication nonadherence resulted in significant improvement in medication adherence, fewer hospitalizations, and fewer mood episodes precipitated by medication nonadherence in a sample of outpatients taking lithium carbonate. Sajatovic and colleagues (2005) also found CBT, interpersonal therapy (ITP), and family-focused treatment (FFT) therapies to be effective in improving treatment adherence. Most cognitive therapies for bipolar disorder involve a multimodal approach. Scott, Garland, and Moorhead (2001) studied the use of one such cognitive therapy as an adjunct to usual psychiatric treatment. The treatment consisted of education, regulation of activities and sleep, stress management, cognitive restructuring, improving medication adherence, and relapse prevention. In the twenty-nine subjects who received cognitive therapy, relapse rates in the eighteen months after commencing treatment showed a 60 percent reduction in comparison with the eighteen months prior to commencing cognitive therapy. Furthermore, 70 percent of subjects who participated viewed cognitive therapy as highly acceptable.

Zaretsky, Segal, and Gemar (1999) studied the effects of cognitive-behavioral therapy on a small sample of patients with either bipolar depression or unipolar depression. Those with bipolar depression achieved similar levels of reduction in depressive symptoms as the unipolar depressed group. However, on measures of more pervasive dysfunctional attitudes, bipolar patients did not improve to the same degree. This finding indicates the need for an approach that targets underlying cognitive and emotional processes. Schema-focused cognitive therapy has been proposed as a way to help bipolar patients reduce cognitive vulnerability to relapse and to adopt effective mood management strategies through attitudinal change (Ball et al., 2003).

Family-focused treatment has been proven successful in improving symptoms of bipolar patients by increasing positive interactions with relatives (Miklowitz et al., 2003; Miklowitz et al., 2000; Simoneau et al., 1999). FFT, not to be confused with a treatment for adjudicated and at-risk youth called functional family therapy, is a time-limited, modularized treatment consisting of psychoeducation, communication enhancement training, and problem-solving skills (Morris, Miklowitz, & Waxmonsky, 2007). According to Miklowitz (2001:533),

The objectives of FFT are to assist the patient and relative in: integrating the experiences associated with mood episodes in bipolar disorder; accepting the notion of a vulnerability to future episodes; accepting a dependency on mood-stabilizing medication for symptom control; distinguishing between the patient's personality and his/her bipolar disorder; recognizing and learning to cope with stressful life events that trigger recurrences of bipolar disorder; and, reestablishing functional relationships after a mood episode.

In the early sessions families are instructed to create a relapse-prevention plan. Information regarding the context of previous episodes and the signs and symptoms that suggest decompensation is discussed, and a document that lists concrete steps for intervening when symptoms increase or worsen is created (Morris, Miklowitz, & Waxmonsky, 2007).

Another treatment approach that has received empirical support is interpersonal and social rhythm therapy. This model is based on the notion that disruptions in the bipolar patient's social rhythms, and eventually circadian rhythms and sleep-wake cycles, will lead to the development of bipolar symptoms. It combines the basic principles of interpersonal psychotherapy with behavioral techniques to help patients regularize their daily routines, diminish interpersonal problems, and adhere to medication regimens (Frank, Swartz, & Kupfer, 2000). Interpersonal and social rhythm therapy has been shown to improve occupational functioning during the acute treatment phase, especially among women (Frank et al., 2008), and to decrease the recurrence of mood episodes during the maintenance phase of treatment (Frank et al., 2005).

Education is another critical component of bipolar treatment. Perry and colleagues (1999) conducted a randomized controlled study of the efficacy of teaching patients with bipolar disorder to identify early symptoms of relapse and to obtain treatment. The patients who received seven to twelve education sessions with routine treatment took a significantly longer time to relapse and had fewer manic episodes in an eighteen-month period than those receiving routine treatment alone. The experimental treatment also improved social functioning and employment, but it had no effect on the recurrence of depressive episodes. Psychoeducation has also been shown to improve relapse rates among bipolar patients with comorbid personality disorders (Colom et al., 2004).

The high suicide rate among individuals with bipolar disorder must be acknowledged. The suicide rate among bipolar persons is approximately twenty times that of the general population (Tondo, Isacsson, & Baldessarini, 2003). Some of the risk factors for suicide include previous suicide attempts or violent acts, previous severe and frequently recurring depression, substance-use comorbidity, current depression or dysphoric-agitated states, hopelessness, current stressors (e.g. loss, separation, medical illness, financial crisis), impulsivity, and ready access to firearms or toxins (Fagiolini et al., 2004; Tondo, Isacsson, & Baldessarini, 2003). Close clinical monitoring; teaching problem-solving skills; rapid hospitalization; the use of medications such as lithium, antipsychotics, or antidepressants; and the various psychosocial interventions are among the strategies used to reduce the occurrence of suicide (Tondo, Isacsson, & Baldessarini, 2003).

The treatment of major depression looks very similar to that of bipolar disorder in that it is often integrative and multimodal. According to Segal, Whitney, and Lam (2001:298), "Psychotherapy for depression is usually taught within the context of discrete treatment modalities . . . practicing clinicians, however, are more likely to use an eclectic mix of strategies from different models." The authors appropriately warn that this approach might "dilute the strategies of a single model." However, clinicians might argue that the use of strategies derived from different models (e.g., cognitive-behavioral and interpersonal) is necessary because of poor responses to a single model, the limited scope of a single model, or complicated presentations requiring multiple and varied strategies, among other things (e.g., lack of resources, time limitation, comorbid issues). Unfortunately, as mentioned previously, the eclectic approach does not lend itself well to outcome studies because of its inherent flexibility.

Cognitive-behavioral therapy and interpersonal therapy have been suggested as first-line treatments of major depression (Parikh et al., 2009). CBT is one of the most well-established treatments for major depression (Parikh et al., 2009) and it continues to advance as researchers and clinicians refine strategies and target specific populations (Kuyken, Dalgleish, & Holden, 2007). The primary goals of CBT are to increase participation in healthy, esteem-building activity and to decrease self-defeating thought processes. ITP has been shown to produce similar outcomes to CBT (Vittengl et al., 2007; Shea et al., 1992; Elkin et al., 1989). Interpersonal therapy focuses more on improving relationships and social skills to reduce stress and vulnerability to relapse.

A recent meta-analysis of the effects of CBT, which involved twenty-eight studies and 1,880 adults, showed that such therapy administered during the acute phase of major depression reduced relapse (or recurrence) significantly compared to pharmacotherapy (Vittengl et al., 2007). Specifically, the researchers claim depressed patients receiving acute cognitive therapy alone or combined with pharmacotherapy have a 61 percent chance of a better outcome (not relapsing or recurring) than a patient treated with pharmacotherapy alone. Other studies provide data that suggest CBT, ITP, and pharmacotherapy demonstrate a similar degree of effectiveness among depressed patients (Bellino et al., 2007; Gloagen et al., 1998; Elkin et al., 1995).

The research comparing depressive treatments among the more severely depressed patients appears inconsistent, and the idea of combining treatments has been controversial (Hegerl, Plattner, & Möller, 2003). The NIMH Treatment of Depression Collaborative Research Program (TDCRP) provided evidence that either drug treatment (imipramine) and case management or interpersonal therapy might produce better initial outcomes than CBT among those with more severe symptomatology (Elkin et al., 1995). On the other hand, DeRubeis and colleagues (1999) conducted a meta-analysis of four major randomized trials and found that there were minimal differences between CBT and antidepressant medication for severely depressed patients, with CBT having a slightly greater effect size. The researchers conclude that empirical evidence does not support the notion that antidepressant medication is superior to cognitive-behavioral therapy for the acute treatment of severely depressed outpatients as suggested by the findings of the TDCRP.

The Coping with Depression (CWD) Course (Lewinsohn et al., 1984) was developed to train depressed adults in several various skill areas, such as increasing levels of pleasurable activity, decreasing depressive thinking, relaxation training, and improving social skills. The participant is taught several different strategies over the course of several weeks and is encouraged to focus on the ones that seem most appropriate to his or her own needs. This educational approach has also received empirical support (Haringsma et al., 2006; Antonuccio, 1998). Reported contraindications of the approach include patients with mental retardation, significant auditory-visual impairment, dyslexia, bipolar disorder, schizophrenia, schizoaffective disorder, or acute substance abuse (Antonuccio et al., 2000).

Sometimes depressed individuals can be difficult to engage in treatment, and the use of motivational interviewing has been proposed as a way to address this issue (Zuckoff, Swartz, & Grote, 2008). When used as an adjunct to other treatments, such as CBT, motivational interviewing may improve retention rates and level of involvement in the treatment process. MI has also been adapted for treating individuals who are suicidal or engage in deliberate self-harm (Zerler, 2008). For this population, an MI approach can promote life-affirming change while encouraging autonomy and self-efficacy, which stands in stark contrast to more common approaches that require the person to involuntarily relinquish all control to the treatment provider.

PTSD AND PANIC DISORDER

Severe anxiety can be debilitating. Symptoms vary from constant worry and fear to physical reactions such as difficulty breathing, stomachache, headache, shaking, dizziness, tension, and sweating. These anxiety symptoms might be generalized, causing constant discomfort, or they might be triggered only in certain situations.

There are several different kinds of anxiety treatments. Some interventions target the biology of the individual while others focus on the person's behavior, thoughts, and social system. The strategies selected are based on the type of illness the individual is experiencing, the level of severity of the condition, and the ability of the individual to engage in treatment.

A review of posttraumatic stress disorder theory and treatment indicates the need for an integrative, multimodal approach to this complicated condition. Wilson (1994) posited that there are five dimensions to an individual's subjective response to trauma: emotional, cognitive, motivational, neurophysiological, and coping resources. Referring to the treatment of PTSD, Shalev and colleagues (2000:374) claimed, "An etiological treatment approach postulates that given the complex psychological, biological, and social abnormalities associated with this disorder, it is not unreasonable to consider different therapeutic approaches to target different symptoms."

Scurfield (1994) suggested an integrative treatment approach that includes stopping retraumatizing behaviors (e.g., substance abuse, excessive thrill seeking, self-destruction), education regarding traumatic stress and recovery, psychiatric medication, symptom management, therapeutic re-experiencing of aspects of trauma, cognitive reframing, facilitation of positive leisure/relationship activities, and addressing spiritual or religious issues, among other things. Eagle (1998) also described an integrative therapy model (Wits trauma intervention model) for individuals experiencing traumatic stress. This model integrates cognitive-behavioral and psychodynamic approaches and includes telling/retelling the story, normalizing the symptoms, addressing self-blame or survivor guilt (restoring self-respect), encouraging mastery, and facilitating creation of meaning.

Posttraumatic stress disorder treatment can be divided into two primary categories: direct therapeutic exposure and anxiety (or stress) management techniques (Hacker Hughes & Thompson, 1994). The anxiety management techniques concentrate on affective, behavioral, and cognitive aspects of PTSD and typically include relaxation training (Livanou, 2001; Miller & DePilato, 1983), breathing retraining (Livanou, 2001), modeling (Livanou, 2001), thought stopping (Livanou, 2001), behavioral rehearsal (Harvard, 1996), cognitive restructuring (Kevan, Gumley, & Coletta, 2007; Thrasher et al., 1996; Harvard, 1996), assertiveness training (Harvard, 1996), education (Meichenbaum, 1974), stress management and coping skills (Anderson & Grunert, 1997; Harvard, 1996) and guided self-dialogue or positive self-statements (Meichenbaum, 1974). Many researchers have offered support for this type of treatment. For instance, Resick and colleagues (1988) found that stress inoculation training, assertion training, and group supportive therapy each produced significant improvements in PTSD symptoms that remained at a six-month follow-up in a sample of sexual assault victims. Kelly and colleagues (2009) demonstrated improvement in multiple areas of PTSD symptomatology following CBT treatment.

Learning skills that facilitate emotion regulation is often considered the most appropriate treatment goal for trauma survivors in the early stage of recovery and for those who are experiencing acute symptomatology (Wolfsdorf & Zlotnik, 2001; Herman, 1992). In a study conducted with a high-risk clinical group of survivors of childhood sexual abuse who presented with PTSD, those who completed an affect-management treatment group reported significantly fewer posttreatment symptoms of PTSD and dissociation than did a wait-list control group (Zlotnick et al., 1997). Material covered in the group sessions included education regarding PTSD, dissociation, flashbacks, "safe" sleep, identification of emotions, crisis planning, anger management, and techniques for distraction, self-soothing, distress tolerance, and relaxation. Skills training in the areas of distress tolerance and emotion regulation make up a large part of the curriculum in Linehan's (1993b) dialectical behavior therapy, and some of the material used in these groups was derived from her work.

Other symptom-management strategies have been suggested. For example, Matsakis (1994) suggested it is typically necessary for the patient to practice adequate physical self-care, create a safe external environment, become able to recognize and learn to cope with and plan for triggers, use anger management strategies, and learn ways to improve sleep, among others. Keane, Street, and Orcutt (2000) described an intervention sequence that began with the client contracting to restrict all alcohol use, followed by a period of psychoeducation about biological, interpersonal, and psychological effects of PTSD. Next, muscle relaxation and deep breathing were taught, followed by several sessions of systematic desensitization that involved elements of the traumatic event. Finally, in vivo exposure completed the treatment sequence.

The PTSD and acute stress disorder (ASD) treatment guidelines suggested by the Australian Center for Posttraumatic Mental Health (ACPMH) include the recommendation that practitioners also focus on vocational, family, and social rehabilitation interventions from the beginning of treatment. Brief eclectic psychotherapy, which includes an emphasis on the patient's partner and work-related problems, has received empirical support for the treatment of PTSD (Lindauer et al., 2005). This treatment combines cognitive-behavioral and psychodynamic approaches and involves writing a letter to persons and institutions related to the trauma throughout treatment and a farewell ritual at the end of treatment.

Motivation is another characteristic of the PTSD client that must be addressed during treatment. While studying outcome predictions among outpatient veterans diagnosed with PTSD, Rooney and colleagues (2007) found that those who have an increased readiness to change and who make more use of behavioral processes of change are likely to have improved outcomes. In other words, individuals who are more committed to change and can successfully substitute healthy behaviors (e.g., relaxation and graduated exposure) for problem behaviors (e.g., avoidance) are expected to have better treatment outcomes.

People develop various levels of resiliency to stressful events, and some individuals who suffer from PTSD might need to increase their resiliency to avoid exacerbating current issues or adding new ones. Kobasa (1979) studied the effects of stressful life events on health in a sample of executives and found that those who experienced significant stress events but had a low incidence of illness following these events have a stronger commitment to self, an attitude of vigorousness toward the environment, a sense of meaningfulness, and an internal locus of control. Some of these characteristics are deeply rooted as part of a person's temperament and personality; however, therapeutic strategies exist that can increase these qualities in people who lack them.

Once the individual begins to establish a sense of emotional equilibrium, cognitive-oriented therapies can be provided. Several studies have demonstrated the effectiveness of cognitive and cognitive-behavioral treatments for various trauma populations, such as sexual assault victims (Foa, Hearst-Ikeda, & Perry, 1995; Nishith et al., 1995; Sharpe, Tarrier, & Rotundo, 1994; Resick & Schnicke, 1992; Foa, Rothbaum, Riggs, & Murdock, 1991; Frank et al., 1988) and combat veterans (Lawson, 1995; McCormack, 1985). Thrasher and colleagues (1996) described the successful treatment of two men with chronic PTSD using cognitive restructuring alone. Thought records were the primary strategy used to challenge dysfunctional cognitions related to shame, self-blame, fear of losing control, and exaggerated perceptions of risk and danger. The treatment was brief, and both short-term and long-term gains were significant. The researchers suggest that cognitive restructuring is an effective alternative for processing traumatic information when exposure is contraindicated. The combination of cognitive restructuring and exposure (imaginal and in vivo) has also been proven effective for the treatment of PTSD (Power et al., 2002). Kevan, Gumley, and Coletta (2007) reported significant treatment gains in a patient with PTSD and comorbid schizophrenia using cognitive restructuring and written elaboration of the trauma memory.

Several pharmacological treatments (e.g., SSRI, monoamine oxidase inhibitors [MAOI], tricyclic antidepressants [TCA]) have also been proven effective for managing PTSD symptoms (Seedat, Stein, & Carey, 2005). However, psychological therapies are generally more beneficial than pharmacotherapies in reducing PTSD symptoms (Van Etten & Taylor, 1998).

After conducting a meta-analysis of the multiple published and unpublished studies on PTSD, both the National Institute of Clinical Excellence (NICE) and the ACPMH suggest there is evidence that trauma-focused psychological treatment produces larger clinical effects than pharmacological treatment does in most people with posttraumatic or acute stress disorder (Forbes et al., 2007; NICE, 2005). However, if the individual is not able to engage in trauma-focused psychological treatment (i.e., is in a crisis state, has severe dissociative symptoms, or has an intellectual or a cognitive disability), then pharmacological interventions are indicated (Forbes et al., 2007).

Panic disorder treatment is similar to the treatment of PTSD in many ways. One of the differences is the emphasis on exposure with panic disorder (First & Tasman, 2005). Meta-analyses by Barlow and colleagues (2005) and Clum, Clum, & Surls (1993) support the effectiveness of exposure, combination treatments (drug and exposure therapies), and psychological coping treatments for panic disorder. Cognitive-behavioral treatment, including cognitive restructuring (Vögele et al., 2010; Margraf et al., 1993; Beck et al., 1992), use of self-coping statements (Waddell, Barlow, & O'Brien,1984), breathing retraining (Meuret, Wilhelm & Roth, 2004; Garssen, de Ruiter, & van Dyck,1992), and progressive muscle relaxation (Barlow et al., 1989), is one of the more popular approaches and has been proven effective in reducing the intensity and frequency of panic attacks.

Combined, or integrated, treatments have also been proven effective for the treatment of panic disorder. Most workbooks and handbooks for treating panic disorder include a variety of cognitive, behavioral, social, and other strategies (Wolfe, 2005; Pollard & Zuercher-White, 2003; Elliott & Smith, 2003; Craske & Barlow, 2001; Zuercher-White, 1997). Following an analysis of the current research, Datillio (2001) suggested a combination of exposure and cognitive-behavioral techniques that promote effective coping for the treatment of panic. Several techniques were recommended for crisis intervention with those experiencing panic disorder: controlled breathing, symptom induction and deescalation, and paradoxical intention. Both short- and long-term gains have been demonstrated with panic inoculation training (panic control treatment), which begins with panic education and cognitive restructuring and proceeds to interoceptive exposure with reattribution of somatic phenomena (Barlow et al., 2000; Klosko et al., 1990; Barlow et al., 1989; Craske, Brown, & Barlow, 1991).

There is also evidence that panic disorder can be effectively treated within a brief treatment context (Otto et al., 2012; Smith 2010). In one study, an intensive, two-day cognitive-behavioral group treatment consisting of education, teaching skills in breathing retraining and cognitive restructuring, in vivo exposure, group discussion, and support for significant others resulted in significant treatment gains with a sample of agoraphobic patients (Evans, Holt, & Oei, 1991). Eighty-five percent of the treated individuals were reportedly symptom-free or symptomatically improved up to one year later. Likewise, Westling and Öst (1999) found that four sessions of cognitive-behavioral treatment of panic disorder with minimal agoraphobic symptomatology produced comparable results in ten to thirteen sessions. Furthermore, the results of a study by Swinson and colleagues (1992) suggest that adding an exposure component to panic disorder treatment may prevent the development of agoraphobia.

Psychopharmacological therapies have also received empirical support (Beamish, Granello, & Belcastro, 2002; Beamish et al., 1996). Tricyclic antidepressants (Bakker, van Balkom, & Spinhoven, 2002; Kahn, McNair, & Lipman, 1986), benzodiazepines (Nadiga, Hensley, & Uhlenhuth, 2003; Clum, Clum, & Surls, 1993), and SSRIs (van Apeldoorn et al., 2008; Nadiga, Hensley, & Uhlenhuth, 2003; Black et al., 1993) have each been found to be effective in managing acute symptoms of panic disorder. However, cognitive therapy has been shown to have lasting effects, whereas drug therapies do not (Nadiga, Hensley, & Uhlenhuth, 2003; Margraf et al., 1993). Unfortunately a relapse of panic episodes often occurs shortly after drug therapy is discontinued (Fyer et al., 1987; Noyes, Caudry, & Domingo, 1986). Therefore a combination of psychotherapy (e.g., CBT) and pharmacotherapy (e.g., SSRI) is typically needed for maximum short- and long-term effects (Fahy et al., 1992; Alexander, 1991).

Many of the treatments described above can be quite intimidating to the client. Through the various exposure and other cognitive and behavioral activities, anxiety sufferers are asked to do exactly what they have been trying their hardest to avoid for months, years, and sometimes decades. Westra and Dozois (2006) provided some evidence that motivational interviewing strategies can promote enhanced involvement in the more active and challenging aspects of CBT. These authors have also provided guidelines for using this approach with anxiety sufferers (Westra & Dozois, 2008).

SUBSTANCE-RELATED DISORDERS

The notion that multiple factors determine behavior is frequently reinforced while clinicians provide care to persons with severe mental illness. The problems such people present with are often complex and there are several different ways to conceptualize them. Substance-related disorders are no exception. Thombs (1999:14) suggests, "Theories on addiction should integrate biological, psychological, and social factors in an effort to explain compulsive substance use." He says that this perspective offers a better account of the research on substance abuse and dependence than do single-factor theories.

Problems related to alcohol and drug use may present the greatest challenge when it comes to determining causal factors and choosing treatment modalities. Min, Biegel, and Johnsen (2005) reviewed characteristics of adults with co-occurring substance and mental disorders as compared to adults with mental illness only in a sample of 1,613 patients who received crisis intervention services. The authors of this study found that the dually diagnosed patients were more likely to be hospitalized, and they claimed that these findings suggest that outpatient mental health services are less well equipped to address a psychiatric crisis when it is accompanied by substance use issues. Mueser (2004:26) states, "Access to a range of different interventions for co-occurring disorders may improve the ability of clinicians to engage and tailor treatment to meet clients' unique needs [and] . . . the available evidence suggests that integrated [mental health and substance use] treatment programs improve outcomes compared with nonintegrated approaches." According to Mueser, motivational interviewing, cognitive-behavioral treatment, and group and family-oriented treatments are all promising interventions for co-occurring conditions.

The literature related to brief treatment of substance abuse is ample, and several different treatment approaches, including many integrated ones, have received empirical support. According to Moyer and Finney (2004:45), "In addition to offering encouragement or advice to change, clinicians providing brief interventions typically help their patients establish goals and provide specific skill building strategies they can use in modifying their drinking behavior." Brief interventions have also been shown to be cost effective (Storer, 2003).

Anxiety and depression may be among the many factors linked to substance use (Kay-Lambkin, Baker, & Lewin, 2004; Mehrabian, 2001), and cognitive-behavioral strategies have been used to address both conditions. For instance, Watt and colleagues (2006) studied the effects of a brief CBT intervention targeting anxiety sensitivity (i.e., fear of arousal-related bodily sensations) in a sample of 221 young adult women with dysfunctional drinking behavior. The intervention included three one-hour group sessions that involved psychoeducation, cognitive restructuring, and physical exercise interoceptive exposure. The CBT condition resulted in a significant reduction in conformity-motivated drinking and emotional-relief expectancies among the high anxiety sensitivity participants. There was also a 50 percent reduction in the proportion of individuals meeting criteria for hazardous alcohol use. According to the authors, the findings suggest alcohol abuse might be effectively prevented among high-risk individuals with a brief CBT approach targeting high anxiety sensitivity, and that anxiety sensitivity may operate as one underlying determinant of dysfunctional drinking behavior (Watt et al., 2006).

In a study that assessed brief treatment outcomes among a sample of 214 regular amphetamine users, abstinence was predicted by participation in two or more one-hour treatment sessions combining MI and CBT (Baker et al., 2005). The intervention also had significant short-term beneficial effects on level of depression, with greater benefits achieved the longer the participant was in treatment. The specific protocol for the four-session CBT intervention was as follows, by session: (1) a motivational interview; (2) teaching progressive muscle relaxation and coping self-talk; (3) controlling thoughts about using amphetamine; and (4) coping with lapses and developing a coping drill to use in high-risk situations.

Marijuana use has also been targeted with brief cognitive-behavioral treatment. For example, Lang, Engelander, & Brooke (2000) used pre- and posttest measures to assess the efficacy of a brief treatment that consisted of a single two-and-a-half-hour assessment and treatment session that included a combination of cognitive, skills training, and educational components designed to highlight what each subject wanted to achieve from the session. The subjects also received a self-help booklet that incorporated CBT principles and provided suggestions, information, and strategies to help control cannabis use. The researchers reported a significant reduction in both frequency and amount of use at the one-month follow-up.

Kay-Lambkin, Baker, and Lewin (2004) proposed a "stepped-care approach to treating co-morbid conditions" based on the current outcome literature. The first step is to perform an assessment, offer feedback, and provide self-help resources. The assessment includes screening of alcohol and other drug use, mental health symptoms, physical symptoms, quality-of-life issues, current stressors, and readiness to change. For those who present with suicide risk, risk to others, or need for urgent medical care, crisis intervention is provided instead of self-care instruction. Step two involves continued assessment and a brief motivational intervention. According to the authors, "Specific components of this intervention include motivational interviewing, cognitive-behavioral coping strategies (high-risk situations, reduce craving, etc.) and relapse prevention. This intervention is designed so that any health professional, with minimal psychological training, could deliver the treatment effectively" (419). If necessary, step three involves assessment and a more intensive intervention provided by a more experienced clinician. Pharmacological and longer, more comprehensive cognitive-behavioral and motivational treatments might be employed at this stage. If other, related issues remain unresolved, such as trauma or relationship issues, further steps are taken to address these specifically.

One of the most common targets of intervention is the individual's level of motivation both to stay in treatment and to stop using substances (Ball et al., 2007; Miller & Rollnick, 2002; Baker et al., 2002; Dunn, DeRoo, & Rivara, 2001). In a review by Miller, Yahne & Tonigan (2003), fourteen of the seventeen random, controlled trials of motivational interviewing among drug-abusing or drug-dependent samples reported positive treatment effects. For example, a study by Rohsenow and colleagues (2004) found that cocaine users with low initial motivation for change benefited from two sessions of motivational interviewing. An interesting finding in this study is that the patients with higher motivation had more cocaine use and alcohol problems after motivation enhancement treatment compared to a meditation-relaxation treatment group. This suggests that an assessment of current level of motivation should be conducted prior to initiating this treatment approach, which is intended for individuals who are ambivalent about changing their behavior.

In a large, randomized, controlled trial, a twenty-minute MI session conducted by addiction peer counselors proved effective in reducing substance use among a sample of cocaine- and heroin-abusing men and women screened in the context of a routine medical visit. Cocaine levels in hair were reduced by 29 percent for the intervention group and only 4 percent for the control group. Similarly, opiate levels were reduced by 25 percent in the intervention group versus 4 percent in the control group. The intervention involved typical MI activities, such as discussion about the gap between real and desired quality of life, the creation of an action plan, and a follow-up phone call, whereas the control group received only a written list of treatment options (Bernstein et al., 2005).

Monti and colleagues (2007) achieved similar results. In their study, participants, who were age 18–24 and were being treated in an emergency department, received either a one-session motivational intervention that included personalized feedback or personalized feedback only; each group also received a telephone call one month and three months after baseline. According to the authors, the motivation treatment participants drank fewer days, had fewer heavy drinking days, and drank fewer drinks per week in the past month at the six-month follow-up, and the gains were maintained at twelve months. A thirty-minute motivation-focused behavioral approach was also shown to be effective in reducing risky behavior associated with hepatitis C virus transmission among a sample of 124 injecting drug users (Tucker et al., 2004).

Coping-skills training is another strategy that has received empirical support. Most substance abuse intervention packages address coping skills in one way or another, including psychoanalytic approaches. When describing the contemporary psychoanalytic approach to treating substance abuse, Thombs (1999:92) states, "The goal of treatment is to build ego strength by helping the person develop the capabilities to cope with the demands of the external world." Cognitive-behavioral, motivational, and family-based approaches also emphasize coping skills.

Rohsenow and colleagues (2004) found that group coping skills training reduced cocaine and alcohol use during follow-up for women and reduced alcohol relapse for men and women. An earlier study also provided support for cocaine-specific coping-skills training as an adjunct to treatment for individuals abusing or dependent on cocaine (Monti et al., 1997). In this study, individual coping-skills training based on a functional analysis of high-risk situations (triggers), which was conducted in either a rural residential substance abuse treatment facility or an urban partial hospital setting, was compared to a control treatment that involved meditation and relaxation training. The clients who received the coping skills treatment had significantly fewer cocaine use days, and the length of their longest binge was significantly shorter at the three-month follow-up period compared to clients in the control condition. The treatment consisted of eight one-hour sessions that included the following modules: (1) explain behavior chains and make a list of client's cocaine use triggers; (2) video on high-risk situations and pitfalls with guided discussion; (3) frustration triggers; (4) anger triggers; (5) other negative feelings; (6) assertiveness skills training; (7) pressure to use (social pressure and handling urges); and (8) enhancing positive moods and events.

Twelve-step groups can also be effective in reducing drug and alcohol use. In a sample of patients undergoing alcohol detoxification, greater Alcoholics Anonymous (AA) and Narcotics Anonymous (NA) attendance was shown to be related to better alcohol use outcomes following detoxification (Kahler et al., 2004). In another study, patients who received an intensive referral to a twelve-step group had better alcohol and drug use outcomes at six months. The intensive referral, or directly linking an individual to a twelve-step group volunteer and encouraging participation, resulted in a greater level of attendance and participation than a standard referral (Timko, DeBenedetti, & Billow, 2006). Knack (2009) has provided guidelines for successfully integrating individual psychotherapy and AA participation.

A meta-analysis of family and couples treatment for substance abuse conducted by Stanton and Shadish (1997) indicates a need to include interventions that target families. Their review suggests that family-based treatments may be more effective than any other treatment modality in reducing substance use for some client populations. The method called A Relational Sequence for Engagement (ARISE) was developed for mobilizing the family and social network to engage substance abusers in treatment; it includes a combination of family systems, motivational, and other approaches (Landau et al., 2000). Many alcoholics and drug users may be cut off from their families, and others do not have living family members; thus this mode of intervention will not be useful for everyone. However, discussion and education about the impact of past and present family dynamics, such as family history of substance use, family attitudes toward drug and alcohol use, and the impact of various family stressors and coping strategies, can be beneficial to most addicts.

In conclusion, the severe mental illness treatment literature lends support to the popular notion that psychiatric problems are determined by multiple factors and therefore require multifaceted treatment plans. Clearly, thoughts, behaviors, environments, levels of motivation, and families are all viable targets for intervention. This text reflects this literature in providing a number of different research-backed approaches. Each tool and technique described in the intervention chapters can be traced to the literature review described above.

In the next chapter, a framework for providing acute psychiatric care for persons with psychotic, mood, anxiety, and substance-related disorders is provided. This acute care approach is consistent with the literature related to integrative and multimodal treatment as well as the severe mental illness outcomes research. Additionally, this approach comprises the four primary stages of intervention that are included in most crisis and brief treatment models.

4

Multimodal Acute Care

AS HOSPITAL DIVERSION PROGRAMS serve greater numbers of severely mentally ill consumers, a practical framework is needed to help providers on all levels offer solid acute mental health care. Those who are entrusted to provide acute mental health care take on a tremendous responsibility, and their work can be very challenging. It is important that they act quickly and use effective strategies that can stabilize the person who is decompensating.

In general, mental health professionals are primarily trained to help clients with the typical symptoms and impairments of their mental illness, and they receive less training in helping them during times of crisis when symptoms are exacerbated (Wiger & Harowski, 2003). Furthermore, many of the interdisciplinary staff of hospital diversion programs are equipped only with nondirective supportive therapy skills (e.g., reflective listening, reframing). This is unfortunate because for some conditions, such as panic disorder with agoraphobia or bipolar disorder, more directive and skilled interventions (e.g., panic control treatment and interpersonal and social rhythm therapy, respectively) have been found to be significantly more effective, even in brief therapy scenarios (Frank et al., 2005, 2008; White & Barlow, 2002). If clinicians do not provide meaningful interventions that directly address issues causing crises, hospitalizations will likely occur. More important, as clinicians become better equipped to provide comprehensive treatment, recovery from mental illness will also become a greater reality for severely mentally ill individuals.

This multimodal approach provides a number of discrete interventions providers can utilize. Additionally, it is a multipronged approach, which more accurately addresses the complex experience many severely mentally ill individuals face. The recovery and multimodal approach effectively addresses coping-skill development, environmental and family issues, and underlying psychological liabilities. In the following section, the leading crisis and brief treatment models that provide a basis for the proposed intervention approach are reviewed. Following this is a discussion of the multimodal acute care approach suggested for use in hospital diversion and other similar programs. The intention is not to provide a formal model that requires strict adherence, but rather to offer a practical framework to organize the actions often required for clinicians to provide effective care in acute care situations.

A REVIEW OF CRISIS AND BRIEF INTERVENTION MODELS

As Callahan (1994) has previously explained, there are many terms such as "emergency" and "crisis" that are used to describe a person's clinical presentation and resulting treatment. Characteristics of a psychiatric emergency typically include one or more of the following: an individual is unable to provide adequate self-care, an individual poses a threat to the safety of others, or the individual poses a threat to his or her own safety. These are the criteria most states use to determine eligibility for inpatient hospitalization. According to Callahan, a crisis is the period in which an individual experiences some level of disequilibrium or is no longer able to cope effectively.

Psychiatric emergencies, which might include a plan to cause self-harm may result from this state of crisis and will require immediate attention. Hospital diversion programs often provide intervention to individuals who present at the crisis level. James and Gilliland (2001:3) offer another way of defining a crisis: "Crisis is a perception or experience of an event or situation as an intolerable difficulty that exceeds the person's current resources and coping mechanisms." This definition reveals an essential goal of crisis intervention—to increase or improve the individual's supportive resources and coping skills.

Some people are more vulnerable to experiencing crises. According to Wiger & Harowski (2003:20), "People with mental illness often live in a state of crisis due to their mental illness. The impairments they suffer result in crises such as job loss, relationship turmoil, prejudice, poverty, abuse, homelessness, loneliness, lack of acceptance in society, confusion, life disruptions due to lengthy treatment, distortion of reality, and more." Severely mentally ill individuals often rely on others to guide them through these challenging experiences, and the better this is done, the less vulnerable they will be to experiencing future crises.

Unfortunately most crisis intervention models are not particularly suited for the common crises experienced by individuals with significant levels of psychiatric disturbance. As Ball and colleagues (2005:10) state, "Crisis in individuals with persistent mental illness is a poorly understood phenomenon for which traditional crisis models do not apply." To better understand the nature of crisis among severely mentally ill individuals, Ball and his colleagues qualitatively studied the experiences of fourteen individuals, most of whom were diagnosed with schizophrenia, who were part of either an assertive community treatment program or another intensive community support program. The results of this study led to the development of a theory of crisis for individuals with severe and persistent mental illness.

The theory proposed by Ball and colleagues includes four major components. First, severely mentally ill individuals have an underlying vulnerability. For instance, constant intrusive voices can trigger a crisis in individuals with schizophrenia. Also, loneliness, poverty, homelessness, poor support, frustration, and other stressors contribute to an underlying vulnerability.

Second, an individual experiences a crisis, which is defined as being overwhelmed and lacking control over the situation or oneself. For the severely mentally ill, crisis episodes are often caused by the exacerbation of symptoms or issues related to their illness rather than external precipitants. The participants in the study reported various circumstances that contributed to feelings of being overwhelmed, such as interpersonal conflict, substance use, sleep disturbance, medication issues, and lack of support.

The third component has to do with the immediate response. Severely mentally ill individuals will either seek help or manage alone. The crisis response often depends on the nature of the crisis and the availability of supports, among other things.

The fourth component, crisis resolution and prevention, includes the activities that facilitate stabilization and increased control. This might include medication changes, hospitalization, increased family and social support, assertive community treatment, increased activity, drug rehabilitation, or any other necessary treatments. This model effectively describes the experience of the individual in crisis, but it does not provide a practical framework for intervention.

James and Gilliland (2001) have offered four crisis intervention models: the equilibrium model, the cognitive model, the psychosocial transition model, and the eclectic model. The equilibrium model focuses on bringing the person to a precrisis level of emotional stability. An effort to establish affective control and reduce disorientation typically constitutes the first phase of intervention. The cognitive model primarily addresses thoughts and beliefs that are the cause of, or contributing factors to, the current crisis state. This intervention is appropriate once the individual has achieved emotional stability and is no longer disoriented. The psychosocial transition model addresses difficulties related to the individual's various systems, such as family, peers, and work. It also focuses on resolving issues related to social supports, finances, shelter, and other external factors that might contribute to the crisis state. Although each of these models addresses important factors, James and Gilliland state that "no strategy applies to every crisis situation" (xvi).

James and Gilliand's fourth model draws from the three models described above. Eclectic crisis intervention theory is based on the premise that the use of a single treatment model is often insufficient, and the use of multiple perspectives and tools is most appropriate. They write, "Eclectic crisis intervention involves intentionally and systematically selecting and integrating valid concepts and strategies from all available approaches to helping clients" (16). These authors promote the use of eclecticism throughout their popular text titled Crisis Intervention Strategies.

In addition to eclectic crisis intervention, there are also brief treatment models that are relevant to the treatment of individuals with severe mental illness. One example comes from Menikoff (1999b:42), who proposed seven principles of behavioral home care:

(1) Establish and maintain a therapeutic alliance; (2) Monitor clinical condition (i.e., ongoing assessment); (3) Educate the patient and significant others; (4) Encourage treatment compliance; (5) Foster structured, fulfilling daily activities; (6) Enhance patient's grasp of the illness, identify new episodes early, and help patient adapt to psychosocial effects of the illness; and (7) Reduce the morbidity and sequelae through the use of community supports.

A PROPOSED ACUTE CARE APPROACH

While attention to practical issues was the primary focus during the development of this text, an attempt was also made to create an intervention approach that is consistent with an emerging paradigm shift in psychological conceptualization and intervention, which will likely have a significant impact on the use and content of treatment manuals (Barlow, 2009). Until recently, treatment protocols have been increasingly narrow in focus, targeting single disorders or symptom clusters. Although this has benefited manual writers, it has not been as helpful for clinicians who do not have time to become proficient with several different protocols (Barlow, 2009). Furthermore, after a review of the many protocols available for anxiety, mood, and other disorders, it becomes evident that there is much overlap in the content of these resources. An alternative to this approach is to develop a unified treatment protocol that can be easily disseminated.

The unified transdiagnostic protocol for the treatment and prevention of emotional disorders developed by Barlow and colleagues at the Center for Anxiety and Related Disorders at Boston University is one such model. These researchers have created a brief treatment protocol based on their extensive research on emotional disorders. The protocol includes various modules such as psychoeducation, emotion regulation strategies, motivational interviewing, thought change strategies, and exposure strategies (Barlow, 2009; Moses & Barlow, 2006). The multimodal acute care approach used in this text is very similar in that it includes several fundamental tools and techniques that can be used with most conditions; however, diagnosis specific strategies are also provided.

The interventions described in this book are multimodal. The recommended techniques are outcome driven, not theory driven; are selected from more than one theoretical orientation, and are drawn from empirically supported treatment protocols. Additionally, the strategies target several aspects of the individual's life. Although using one particular theory as a guide is not the priority, the multimodal acute care approach fits neatly within the frameworks of social-learning and cognitive-behavioral theories.

Acute psychiatric or crisis care providers do not enjoy the luxury of time that outpatient psychotherapy often affords. Acute care must be approached with more flexibility and a willingness to consider multiple intervention strategies because the time is limited. Additionally, the decompensating person benefits more from an intervention that he or she is comfortable with and willing to engage in; therefore treatment providers need to be accommodating and have a variety of strategies at their disposal.

An example of the need for an eclectic and multimodal approach can be seen in the treatment of panic disorder with agoraphobia. The intense anxiety and fear that is characteristic of this disorder can be targeted in many ways because usually many behaviors (avoidance), thoughts (I'm going to die), and interpersonal patterns (selecting enabling partners) are involved. Cognitive-behavioral treatment strategies that involve modifying unhealthy behavioral and thought patterns will be useful in addressing many contributors to the symptoms. However, other factors, such as critical family members, friends, or partners, might also be contributing to the problem. Even if the person learns to challenge negative thoughts, he or she may not achieve significant relief until the environment is significantly changed. In this case, a combination of CBT and interpersonal strategies will likely produce the best results. In this text one will find the integration of cognitive-behavioral, solution-focused, systems, interpersonal, and other therapies.

There is a paucity of literature providing us with evidence-based psychosocial approaches to treating severely mentally ill persons during an acute phase of their illness. An approach that considers the particular resources and limitations of hospital diversion programs is even harder to come by. Therefore multiple sources of literature that directly relate to this particular treatment population (SMI), treatment modality (hospital diversion), and stage of treatment (acute care) have been reviewed and integrated into one practical framework. The resulting multimodal acute care approach is described below.

THEORETICAL BASIS OF THE APPROACH

The multimodal acute care approach was adapted from multimodal therapy (Lazarus, 1981, 1989). MMT is the framework selected for this text because it is designed to be both comprehensive and brief. It also maintains a level of flexibility that many models do not afford. As Lazarus (1997:68) states, "The MMT format presents a versatile and flexible modus operandi for effecting widespread changes and provides both novices and experienced clinicians with an ongoing 'blueprint' for selecting techniques and styles that best suit the needs of individual clients." Furthermore, it does not require an in-depth understanding of complicated theory, nor does it suggest the use of techniques that only experts can successfully perform. Instead, MMT is a practical yet sophisticated approach to treating individuals with mental health concerns that emphasizes efficiency and effectiveness. Lazarus (1997:126) puts it the following way: "Whereas many professionals remain impressed by books and concepts that are complex and indeterminate, if not incomprehensible, my view is that any clinical approach that is not easy to understand, easy to remember, and easy to apply is unworthy of serious attention."

The multimodal acute care approach also borrows heavily from Beutler's systematic treatment selection model. This approach is integrative in that it is open to the use of multiple perspectives, multimodal in that it accounts for the multiple factors that contribute to mental illness, and systematic because interventions are designed for specific purposes, patients, and conditions. The multimodal acute care approach is integrative and multimodal, and the interventions are selected for addressing the acute symptomatology of specific SMI populations.

This integrative approach is advantageous in brief treatment settings where quick and accurate decision making is essential. The notion of matching interventions based on client characteristics seems even more relevant to situations in which individuals are experiencing acute psychiatric illness. If treatment providers learn a set of interventions for not only particular disorders but also specific client characteristics, the time it takes to stabilize an individual should improve. This is most important when speedy and effective intervention can prevent significant negative consequences.

A RECOVERY-ORIENTED APPROACH

"Recovery" is the current paradigm in the field of mental health care. It is primarily a philosophy and an attitude concerning the potential for personal growth and quality of life for individuals with severe mental illness. Mary Ellen Copeland (2007), a pioneer in the recovery movement, states:

> The recovery and self-help skills are meant to compliment other treatments for psychiatric symptoms. Specifically, they are used to promote higher levels of wellness, stability and quality of life; decrease the need for costly,

invasive therapies; decrease the incidence of severe symptoms; decrease traumatic life events caused by severe symptoms; raise client's level of hope and encourage their actively working toward wellness; and increase the client's sense of personal responsibility and empowerment.

Recovery requires the individual who is afflicted by mental illness to learn ways to overcome, not just cope with, a disability (Corrigan & Ralph, 2005).

A recovery approach to hospital diversion involves preparing members of the multidisciplinary treatment teams to provide psychoeducation and brief therapeutic interventions. If each contact with the client is bolstered by an increased therapeutic dynamic, the individual will grow closer to recovery. Menikoff (1999:xxi) suggests that behavioral home care (i.e., ACT) for the mentally ill should encompass "a fluid set of interventions specifically tailored to individual clients and individual situations" where "clients are supported over the immediate crisis, are educated about their illness, and are provided ongoing supports designed to achieve maximum recovery and reintegration into the life of their community." Furthermore, symptom frequency and severity, as well as hospital use, should decrease as program staff are better able to intervene as clients experience relapse or decompensation. Although the primary therapy provider in these programs is the clinical social worker or psychologist, it is common for all team members to be in a position that requires counseling intervention. If each member of a treatment team is capable of reinforcing the therapeutic activities, stabilization will occur more quickly.

There is recent evidence of a push to increase and improve the provision of psychotherapeutic services among assertive community treatment and other hospital diversion programs. For instance, Reynolds and colleagues (2007) provided a chapter on the integration of dialectical behavior therapy into assertive community treatment in Dialectical Behavior Therapy in Clinical Practice: Applications Across Disorders and Settings. Also, Randall and Finkelstein (2007) recently offered a description of how to incorporate cognitive-behavioral therapy into psychiatric rehabilitation day programming (i.e., partial hospitalization).

Previous efforts to train the mental health professional workforce in more clinically focused interventions, such as CBT, have been successful (Tarrier et al., 1999). Two training centers effectively trained community psychiatric nurses to provide psychosocial interventions including case management, family treatment, and cognitive-behavioral treatment. The training resulted in increased knowledge and skills among staff and improvement in functioning among patients treated (Lancashire et al., 1997). This study provides evidence that psychosocial interventions can be used by nonclinical staff within typical community mental health services.

COMPONENTS OF MULTIMODAL ACUTE CARE

The multimodal acute care approach consists of a variety of intervention strategies that are provided within the PEAR framework. This acronym is used to help you remember the stages. It is typically best to follow the Perform assessment → Establish equilibrium → Address social and environmental issues → Relapse prevention progression during the intervention, but it may be necessary to jump steps depending on the individual's needs. The PEAR intervention phases are described below.

Perform assessment. In the assessment phase, the interventionist performs a brief psychosocial assessment. The goal of this assessment is to get enough information to be able to effectively address the individual's immediate needs. The level of assessment depends on the type of program the individual is in. For example, if he or she has been involved in an ACT team the assessment will be shorter because the person is known; if the person is a referral to a crisis stabilization program, a more thorough assessment is typically indicated.

One of the main goals of the assessment is to determine where to start with treatment. Maslow (1970) suggested that unless lower-level needs (e.g., establishing a safe environment) have been met, people are often not concerned with higher-level needs (e.g., self-esteem). Therefore treatment will likely fail if a lower-level need has been skipped. Maslow's hierarchy of needs begins with physiological needs and proceeds to safety, love and belonging, self-esteem, and self-actualization needs.

Establish equilibrium. The treatment phase of the model generally begins with behavioral strategies and includes various steps to establish emotional equilibrium. The literature suggests that teaching various coping or stress management strategies is essential to the treatment of nearly every clinical condition, especially during an acute phase of the illness (Rohsenow et al., 2004; Livanou, 2001; Anderson & Grunert, 1997; Zlotnick et al., 1997;

Harvard, 1996; Herman, 1992; Miller & DePilato, 1983). The task of establishing affective stability often requires the clinician to help the individual who is decompensating to build structure into the day. It is common for individuals with severe mental illness to be lethargic and to feel like each day is the same because of inactivity (Menikoff, 1999b). The lack of daily goals and activities can result in a destructive cycle of inactivity, emptiness, and vulnerability. Something as simple as daily medication monitoring can provide needed structure and a means to gauge the beginning and ending of days. Significant gains can be made if therapeutic activities are scheduled throughout the week, such as visiting friends, going to a clubhouse program, doing volunteer work, or going to a library. A clinic-based program usually provides structure through a consistent daily schedule that includes mealtime, medication administration, group therapy, and individual sessions with counselors. Other strategies, such as improving medication adherence and teaching coping skills, are also used during this phase of intervention.

Address social and environmental issues. The next step is to address systemic problems, such as family issues or other environmental issues that might be exacerbating symptoms or causing significant distress. The need to effectively treat issues related to family and interpersonal problems has been well documented among the target populations of this text (Miklowitz et al., 2003; Barrowclough et al., 2001; Miklowitz et al., 2000; Falloon et al., 1999; Miller & Mason, 1999; Simoneau et al., 1999; Doane et al., 1986). For home-based programs this might include helping family members learn how to better cope with their mentally ill relative. In center-based programs staff might process the frustration of living in a stressful environment and explore housing options with the client. Also staff might help the client problem-solve ways to effectively end abusive or otherwise unhealthy relationships.

Relapse prevention. The final stage targets relapse and attempts to prepare the client for long-term stability. This includes motivational interviewing, cognitive restructuring by way of thought records, establishing participation in a support group, or other activities that will help the individual maintain stability and avoid the need for a higher level of care in the future. Motivational interviewing has been adapted for use with most clinical populations (McCracken & Corrigan, 2008; Zuckoff, Swartz, & Grote, 2008; Zerler, 2008; Westra & Dozois, 2008; Monti et al., 2007) and cognitive-behavioral therapies have been shown to produce both short-term and long-term gains with severely mentally ill clients (Parikh et al., 2009; Kevan, Gumley, & Coletta, 2007; Bechdolf, 2005; Scott, Garland, & Moorhead, 2001; Tarrier et al., 1998; Cochran, 1984; Zaretsky, Segal, & Gemar, 1999; Thrasher et al., 1996; Harvard, 1996; Margraf et al., 1993). The particular tools used in this phase will depend highly on the client's intellectual ability, disorder, and level of participation in the treatment process. The ultimate goal is to take the crisis intervention one step further than immediate relief and to prepare the individual for future success and eventually recovery.

The remaining chapters include the actual intervention strategies. First, the fundamental skills that are relevant to the treatment of all conditions discussed in this text are described. In the chapters that follow, specific issues are addressed for individuals with the most common conditions seen among hospital diversion program clients. Case examples are used to guide treatment providers through the steps of the multimodal acute care approach. Various issues that need to be considered when conducting acute psychiatric treatment are discussed in the final chapter. It will be helpful to first become familiar with the fundamental tools and techniques and then follow the diagnosis-specific protocols as needed to assist clients who need an extra level of care.

5

Fundamental Tools and Techniques

THERE ARE FUNDAMENTAL TOOLS AND TECHNIQUES that can be used in the treatment of most conditions encountered by staff working in hospital diversion programs. These activities, which include various screenings, therapy techniques, and action plans, comprise the core intervention sequence for this text. Other, more diagnosis-specific, interventions will be discussed in the following chapters. The interventions are described below in the order they would typically be used during the course of treatment.

As mentioned earlier, it is important to treat clients at a level that is appropriately aligned with one's training and experience. Table 5.1 provides guidance on which interventions to use. This guide includes beginner, intermediate, and advanced levels of clinical competence, which are represented by one, two, or three asterisks. Every tool or technique has been assigned a particular difficulty level.

SUICIDE/SELF-HARM ASSESSMENT*

Establishing safety is the priority when treating the client who presents with acute care needs. It is essential to assess whether the individual's acute symptomatology includes thoughts of self-harm, especially if the person has a known history of suicidal behavior. Joiner (2005) proposes a model of suicide that requires a person to have three characteristics for successful death by suicide: (1) an acquired ability to enact lethal self-injury (e.g., through previous self-injury and suicide attempts; a history of abuse, vio-

TABLE 5.1 Intervention Difficulty Guide

DIFFICULTY LEVEL	COMPETENCY
*Beginner**	Requires basic counseling skills, such as empathic listening, problem solving, and effective communication.
*Intermediate***	Requires more formal training and experience in specific counseling techniques, and often a more comprehensive understanding of the specific theoretical framework. The ability to successfully and safely process emotions with the client is essential.
*Advanced****	Should only be performed by a trained clinician who is capable of effectively responding to strong emotional reactions and complicated clinical scenarios.

lence, or significant injury; an increased pain tolerance); (2) the feeling that one does not belong (i.e., feeling disconnected, lonely, outcast); (3) the belief that one is a burden and others would be better off in one's absence. All clients should be monitored for suicide or self-harm behavior, but those who match these characteristics will need to have specific goals related to suicide and self-harm included in their treatment plan.

Self-injury and self-mutilation, such as cutting, are often recognizable, but sometimes there are no clues to suggest a client engages in these behaviors. Therefore it is important to inquire about this during the assessment. Do not be afraid to ask clients if they have had thoughts of self-harm and if they have had thoughts of ending their life (two distinct questions). If they say yes to either, ask when these thoughts occurred. If the thoughts are recent or current, ask if they have a specific plan. If they have a plan, ask what the likelihood is that they might try it. Also try to determine if they have the means to carry out the plan. If the person seems ambivalent about self-harm, attempt to get him or her to contract for safety. A verbal contract is acceptable, but a written one is preferred (see below for details). If the person is unable to contract for safety, necessary steps should be taken to try to secure inpatient care or some other form of twenty-four-hour monitoring.

Self-harm behavior is more common among individuals who have experienced significant trauma. For this reason and others, it is important to ask the client about the presence of traumatic events in his or her lifetime.

For example, one might ask: Have you ever been or are you currently being physically or sexually abused? Have you been abused in any other way? Have you witnessed or experienced anything that was traumatic (i.e., significantly painful, hurtful, disturbing, or causing nightmares or flashbacks)? Furthermore, there are several reasons why individuals engage in self-harm behavior, and it will be helpful to find out why the client does this. Common reasons include to control feelings, to experience feelings because the person has numbed his or her emotions, to prove to others that one is in pain, to express overwhelming emotional pain as physical pain is more tolerable than emotional pain, and to punish people.

Treatment providers should offer other, healthier, ways to achieve the same goal the client is trying to achieve through self-injury. For instance, if clients are cutting because they need to feel physical pain, one could suggest that they hold ice cubes to feel the pain. They will likely say that the new strategy just is not the same, but continue to encourage them. Try explaining that there are fewer negative consequences when they use the healthy coping alternatives.

A second measure that is often necessary, and could be included in a safety contract, is to remove all objects that could be used for violence from the home. Until various symptoms such as extreme emotionality and impulsivity can be effectively addressed, safe-proofing the home and environment is the best way to reduce the potential for harm. This might include removing specific objects or people that trigger stress reactions or exacerbate negative emotions, as well as items around the home that present an opportunity for harm to self or others. Objects that would likely need to be removed include guns, knives, razors, ropes or chords, medications (give only what is needed each day), alcohol, various tools, or anything else that could cause significant harm. Some individuals may need to turnover their car keys, especially if they have ever had an urge to wreck their car during times of high stress.

If the client is currently enduring trauma, such as physical abuse, this issue should be properly addressed. If it appears that mood, anxiety, or psychotic symptoms are connected to past or recent trauma (i.e., the client has comorbid PTSD), then treatment will likely need to include relevant PTSD strategies (discussed in chapter 8). Whether a history of trauma is identified, clients who engage in self-harm are in need of immediate attention. They are trying to manage symptoms in a way that works for them, and they need to be introduced to new, safer skills before the potential for severe injury, and death, becomes any greater.

DRUG SCREEN*

Even if the individual being treated has never been known to use substances, it is still a good idea to explore this as a possible contributor to the current crisis. However, this assessment needs to be performed cautiously so that the individual does not feel disrespected or distrusted. It may be helpful to use a drug detection instrument such as a breathalyzer or urine drug screen to determine which substances are being used. Some clients may be more willing to admit to using some substances but not others, and some of these instruments can help verify or correct reported amounts of substance use. These assessments are easier to conduct when they are part of a standard protocol because clients will be less likely to feel singled out or distrusted. Clinicians can also remind clients that it is understood that their difficulties are real and that they truly want to help them. Drug screens can also be used to monitor compliance with contracts as well as the effectiveness of the intervention.

More practically, there are several quick questionnaires available for assessing specific substance use behaviors and consequences. The CAGE questionnaire (Ewing, 1984) and Drug Abuse Screening Test (Skinner, 1982) have been shown to have clinical utility with the SMI population (Maisto et al., 2000). Items cover the specific information necessary for determining DSM-IV diagnoses and can help facilitate treatment planning.

CAGE QUESTIONNAIRE

Instructor: Ask each question. Two "yes" responses indicate that the possibility of alcoholism should be investigated further

1. Have you ever felt you should cut down on your drinking? Yes / No
2. Have people annoyed you by criticizing your drinking? Yes / No
3. Have you ever felt bad or guilty about your drinking? Yes / No
4. Have you ever had a drink first thing in the morning to steady your nerves or get rid of a hangover (eye-opener)? Yes / No

DAST-10

Instructions: These questions refer to the past twelve months. "Drug abuse" refers to the use of prescribed or over-the-counter drugs in excess of the directions and any nonmedical use of drugs. The questions do not include alcoholic beverages.

Circle Your Response

1. Have you used drugs other than those required for medical reasons? Yes / No
2. Do you abuse more than one drug at a time? Yes / No
3. Are you always able to stop using drugs when you want to? Yes / No
4. Have you had "blackouts" or "flashbacks" as a result of drug use? Yes / No
5. Do you ever feel bad or guilty about your drug use? Yes / No
6. Does your spouse (or parents) ever complain about your involvement with drugs? Yes / No
7. Have you neglected your family because of your use of drugs? Yes / No
8. Have you engaged in illegal activities in order to obtain drugs? Yes / No
9. Have you ever experienced withdrawal symptoms (felt sick) when you stopped taking drugs? Yes / No
10. Have you had medical problems as a result of your drug use (e.g., memory loss, hepatitis, convulsions, bleeding)? Yes / No

Scoring / Interpretation: Score 1 point for each question answered "yes," except for question 3, for which a "no" receives 1 point. A score of 0 indicates no reported problems; 1–2 indicates a low degree of problems; 3–5 indicates a moderate degree of problems.

If it is discovered that the client is currently using substances, he or she should be encouraged to contract to stay alcohol and drug free during treatment. If detoxification is necessary, a referral to a medical treatment center should be made before beginning other interventions. It is not uncommon for severely mentally ill clients to self-medicate with alcohol, marijuana, or other substances. They need to know that substance use can be an impediment to the intervention process and that it is unlikely that their psychiatric health will stabilize until they cease these activities. Clients who are using should be provided education regarding the potentially life-threatening effects of combining alcohol and some psychotropic medications, such as benzodiazepines, as well as the effects street drugs can have on the efficacy of prescription medications.

Substance use and withdrawal from substances can cause symptoms that mimic depressive, panic, manic, and psychotic symptoms. This makes it difficult to determine if the symptoms triggered the substance use or if the substance use triggered the symptoms. The cyclical nature of substance use indicates a need to treat both conditions simultaneously.

CRISIS ACTION PLAN*

The crisis action plan (see appendix A) is a client's blueprint for achieving stability. It is best to complete the action plan with the individual in crisis when he or she can tolerate answering several questions. This worksheet allows the clinician to obtain information about the individual's symptoms, triggers, and treatment preferences. It also gives the clinician an opportunity to learn about the coping strategies that have been effective in the past, as well as ones to avoid, and it gives the client strategies to implement immediately.

CONTRACTS*

One of the first things that can be done to reduce risk of self-harm, violence, or intoxication is to establish a safety contract. Williams (1994:168–69) writes:

> Contracts between client and therapist help the client feel safe from self-destructive thoughts, impulses, or actions and to have alternatives should he or she become out of control-other contracts between client and therapist or therapist, client, and the client's family can determine when hospitalization needs to be considered and where it should occur.

It can be helpful for the person in crisis to have clear direction and to feel a sense of commitment to becoming well again. Contracts, both verbal and written, will sometimes provide just enough of a sense of commitment to prevent the client from engaging in self-harm or other destructive behavior, such as substance use. Also, a client's willingness or unwillingness to contract for safety may help clinicians determine whether or not to refer the client to a more restrictive level of care. Contracts do not provide a guarantee of safety or compliance; thus ongoing suicide and self-harm assessment and interventions that address suicidal behavior should not end with the contract. Contracting should be conducted as a supportive action rather than a punitive one. For example, clinicians can say, "I want to give you some extra help with your commitment to treatment by having you sign this contract with me" versus "You have to sign this contract and if you violate it . . . you will have to leave the program . . . I will call your . . . you can no longer . . . ." Clinicians can have the client sign new contracts daily or weekly if it is necessary to reinforce the client's commitment.

IMPROVE COPING SKILLS*

The individual in crisis will likely need to be taught additional coping strategies. Dialectical behavior therapy, developed by Marsha Linehan, includes "crisis survival strategies" that help the individual cope with the present moment of significant distress (Linehan, 1993b). Writers in the area of anxiety and panic have also suggested strategies that parallel Linehan's (Elliott & Smith, 2003). The typical strategies include distracting the mind from negativity and symptom triggers through activities such as exercise, walking, cleaning, helping others, books, movies, working on a puzzle, watching TV, counting, or hot/cold showers; soothing the senses by looking at pleasant pictures, listening to music, observing silence, lighting a scented candle, taking a warm bath/shower, or enjoying a favorite food/drink; and trying to make the stressful moment more tolerable through positive imagery, making meaning out of the situation, prayer, relaxation strategies, focusing on one thing at a time, and positive, encouraging self-talk.

Becoming skillful at these activities will increase the likelihood of successfully becoming less distressed. The key is to find a few of these strategies that work well for the individual in crisis and add them to the strategies he or she has used successfully in the past. Also, encourage clients to practice the coping strategies to make them more effective and to continue to use them as needed. Many times clients have skills that they regularly use but might not be aware of. Asking them "What are three things you do to help yourself feel better?" can be a good way of making them aware of skills they already regularly use. Some other things that might help reduce overall distress are as follows:

- Advise clients to avoid stimulants that might worsen anxiety, like coffee, caffeine, and large amounts of sugar.
- Some clients will benefit from some kind of exercise or physical activity. If the individual can tolerate a gradual increase in exercise (e.g., walking, stretching, biking, aerobics) and is in good physical health, encourage him or her to try this.
- Encourage good sleep hygiene. This includes making the bedroom environment comfortable (cool, quiet, dark), exercising in the afternoon, taking a relaxing bath or shower before going to bed, establishing a regular pattern of sleep, avoiding daytime naps, and avoiding eating heavy foods and drinking caffeinated beverages before bedtime (Van Brunt & Lichstein, 2000).
- Many individuals with severe mental illness smoke excessively and may become anxious if they do not have their regular dose of nicotine. So it is important to find out if some of their anxiety is related to being out of cigarettes. If this is the case, and they have no desire to quit smoking, it might be helpful to assist them in obtaining cigarettes to help them through the crisis. They should also be encouraged to budget their cigarettes appropriately so that they do not run out in the future.

ACTIVITY SCHEDULING*

In many cases inactivity will cause boredom, depression, physical health problems, and other issues that can exacerbate symptoms. Therefore an effort to increase socialization and physical activity can be an important part of the integrative treatment. The first step in increasing activity is to create a pleasurable activities checklist. Have the client think about the things he or she likes to do (e.g., walking, talking with friends or family, going to the park, watching action movies, cooking) and then write them down on a piece of paper. Next, go through the list and discuss specific ways to begin incorporating these activities into a daily schedule. It is important that a realistic plan is developed and that the necessary supports are in place to prevent failed attempts, which could exacerbate depression or decrease motivation for future efforts. Many clients, especially those with limited resources, will need a substantial amount of help in generating activities that they can begin doing.

The second aspect of activity scheduling is to create a daily activity log. This journal of attempted activities will provide accountability as well as a way to monitor which activities are helpful in improving the client's mood. If the client is having trouble engaging in the selected activities, it is important to quickly generate a new list or address the hurdles preventing participation. For clients who are not able to write or have cognitive impairments, it may be necessary to keep the log for them.

ASSERTIVENESS TRAINING*

Improving assertiveness can have many benefits, such as reduced stress and increased self-esteem and respect from others. Assertiveness training is necessary for those who feel a general lack of control or power. It involves helping the person understand his or her rights and role-playing assertive responses to common scenarios. The goal is to help the client clearly articulate needs and wishes and defend his or her opinion or preference without becoming aggressive.

Assertiveness skills can be enhanced by teaching clients how to identify problems in a situation, to identify thoughts and feelings about the problem, and to express this clearly with short, clear statements. For example, "I know that you feel [other's desire], but I still want [their desire]." Additionally, clinicians can teach clients to use assertive body language. This includes maintaining direct eye contact, having an alert but relaxed posture, and using a calm but serious tone.

MEDICATION ADHERENCE*

It is important to gather information about the individual's current medication use. In some cases a psychotic or mood episode may be the result of a recent medication change. At other times it may be the result of an individual's decision to cease taking medications without proper titration. Another issue could be that the individual is not taking medication properly (e.g., consistently or at the correct time).

If a client has been prescribed psychotropic medication but has not been taking it, find out why. If the client claims to have run out, provide assistance in getting a new prescription. If the client says it does not work, try to determine if it is being taken correctly. If the client says it makes him or her worse, do not ignore this, as many individuals do not respond well to medication. After this information has been gathered, consult with the prescribing physician to find out what to do next.

If there is no reason to suspect that the increased symptoms are a side effect of the medication, the individual will usually be encouraged to continue taking the medication. For instance, if a client was recently discharged from the hospital and has just begun a new medication regimen, it could take time before the medication is effective. It is helpful to document a timeline of medication use and reported symptoms. Consultation with the individual's prescribing physician is a must.

Strategies for increasing medication adherence are as follows:

- Have the client correctly describe each medication.
- Have the client habitually and honestly describe adherence to the medication regimen, and check the report with the pill bottles or pill box.
- Ask the client if there are any reasons not to take the medication, and explore the answers with the client.
- Help the client understand the common error of thinking one can stop medication because one is feeling better or has no symptoms.
- If the client has a history of stopping medication while using alcohol, provide information them about which medications will have a harmful interaction and which will not (consult with a physician).
- Talk with the client about the many important reasons to stay drug and alcohol free.

If these strategies are ineffective, it might be necessary to spend more time on the client's motivation to make necessary changes in his or her life. See the motivation enhancement section below for assistance with this strategy.

GENERAL TIPS FOR ADDRESSING SOCIAL AND ENVIRONMENTAL ISSUES[*]

Many times environmental stress is preventing the client from stabilizing fully or is causing relapse of crisis episodes. Some of the things that might help improve the client's social or environmental situation include:

- Addressing any threats that might be contributing to anxiety and stress
- Decreasing the number of demands on the individual if this is a problem
- Dealing with people who might be trying to sabotage the treatment process
- Increasing positive activities or interactions with family, church, and community
- Making any necessary changes in the individual's current system (peers, family, occupation, community) that might be causing difficulties
- Linking the individual to proper resources for food, clothing, or shelter if needed (e.g., salvation army, abused women's shelter, food pantry, various church missions)

If the client gives permission, and if he or she has supportive family members, it will likely be helpful to include the family in the intervention process. The individual in crisis will likely benefit from having those around him or her be more knowledgeable and sympathetic to difficulties the client is experiencing. Furthermore, the family can act as cotherapist, within reason, by reinforcing the strategies that the individual has been learning. Family and friends need to know what exacerbates the client's symptoms, and the interventionist can empower them to change their manner of responding to the individual, if necessary.

Increase Internal Locus of Control*

The concept of locus of control (LOC) refers to a person's tendency to attribute the things that happen in life to personal (internal) versus environmental (external) causes. Internal factors include things like intelligence, personality, and attitude. External factors include chance, fate, and the influence of others. At least one study has shown that an external locus of control is related to neuroticism, low subjective well-being, low conscientiousness, and low agreeableness (Morrison, 1997). An internal locus of control may protect against illness following stressful life events (Kobasa, 1979). Therefore it might be important to help individuals in crisis strengthen the belief that they can in fact influence what happens to them. Another reason for helping a client develop a more internal locus of control concerns the prediction of change. Individuals who have an internal locus of control will more often accept assistance in changing behavior because they believe their behavior is controllable (Cauce, Hannan, & Sargeant, 1992).

Clinicians can help individuals develop a more internal locus of control by helping them become aware of times that they are exerting their own control over a situation. The intervention provider can also assist clients in writing a list of things they have done to influence aspects of their life and what things they might do to influence it in the future. Clinicians can also have clients write or verbalize empowering self-statements that remind them that they are not powerless and can make changes in their life. The goal is not significant personality change; rather the hope is that individuals will increase their belief that they can effectively make changes in their life and improve their condition. The thought change worksheet (described below) can also be used to change one's beliefs about control.

Motivation Enhancement**

Many individuals with severe mental illness are difficult to engage in the treatment process. This could be due to issues of trust, failed attempts at recovery, and denial of problems, among other things. If clinicians find that they are trying much harder to achieve goals than the client, they likely need to change gears a bit and use motivational interviewing strategies. Not only will this make the current intervention easier and more effective, it will also help sustain the person's dedication to make changes in life and continue the treatment process after the acute episode is over.

Furthermore, one of the primary goals of substance abuse treatment is to encourage commitment to making necessary changes. It can be very difficult to combat the urge to use the drug one is addicted to; therefore motivation must remain high. Through motivational interviewing (Miller & Rollnick, 2002), clients will explore the ambivalence they experience regarding change, improve their commitment to the change process, and become better prepared to take maximum advantage of treatment. The interview typically includes the following activities:

• Identify short-term and long-term life goals. Ask the client to think about and name their short-term goals (for treatment, health, work, etc.) as well as their long-term goals. This task can be difficult for some, and it may illicit strong emotions. More often it can strengthen the therapeutic alliance and will provide a jumping-off point for the other activities.

• Explore importance and confidence. Ask the individual how important it is to make changes in life. For example, "On a scale of 1–10, with 10 being the greatest importance, how important is it for you to be able to make those changes?" If the individual does not feel that this change is important, then treatment should begin with facilitating an exploration of whether the client genuinely enjoys his or her current state. Most times the answer is no. Another tactic involves helping clients see the benefits in making the proposed changes. If possible, provide examples of times that the client has stated he or she is tired of the way things are, and times he or she wishes the situation was different.

Next, ask how confident the client is in the ability to make the desired changes. For example, "On a scale of 1–10, with 10 being the most confident, how confident are you that you can eventually make the changes you are proposing to make?" If the individual gives a low number, it will be necessary to spend some time building a sense of self-confidence so that the person will be willing to engage in the treatment process and to prevent premature cessation of the treatment relationship. Clinicians can do this by pointing to things in the past that the individual has successfully changed or overcome, by building supports, and by providing encouragement.

• Explore values. Engage the client in an exploration of his or her values. A focus on values may stimulate motivation for change. Focusing on discrepancies between ideal life conditions and actual conditions may induce a desire to alter daily behaviors so that they are more congruent with strong beliefs. Ask the individual, "What are some of the things you really value a lot in life?" "Are there any conflicts between your current behaviors or difficulties and the things you value or the things you believe in?" "How can we make your actions more congruent with your values?"

• Look forward. In this exercise have the client envision two futures. Ask the person, "If you continue on the same path without any changes, how will things be five or ten years from now?" Explore the answer with the client, and respectfully challenge any unrealistic thinking. Next ask, "If you make significant changes in the way you manage your symptoms, how will things be five or ten years from now?" The interventionist should focus on eliciting information and encouraging the person to process these questions while avoiding arguing for one side or the other. Clients will not be ready to engage in what could be a difficult treatment process if they do not decide for themselves that they want to make a change.

• Revisit the crisis action plan. If the client has not already identified several ways to use various resources for developing mental health stability and (if necessary) sobriety, help with the completion of this task. Also, integrate as much of the "change talk" that clients have used during the motivation enhancement discussions into the plan. For instance, under the "what I need to do" and "notes" sections, have clients list any new strategies they have learned as well as motivating statements such as "Remember that taking my medications regularly and staying active will help me achieve [insert goal here]" or "I am confident that I can develop a sober lifestyle."

Change Dysfunctional Thinking**

The thought change worksheet (see appendix B) assists the client in challenging maladaptive thoughts and increasing healthy ones. A certain level of emotional stability should be achieved before engaging in cognitive therapy. Also, if the client's intellectual ability is low, or if there is significant cognitive impairment, this strategy will probably have little effect.

The first step is to identify the situation or event that is precipitating distress. This might include having to take medication, paranoia, family conflict, or problems in social environments that are related to symptoms. Next, identify the specific emotional reaction to the stressor. Assist the individual in identifying the specific feelings that are provoked so that he or she can better communicate feelings to others and better track the ability to manage symptoms. In the third column help the client identify the thoughts that automatically come to mind during the panic attack or psychotic or mood episodes. The thoughts "I'm going to die," "Everybody wants to hurt me," and "I am a complete failure" are common examples.

In the next two columns assist clients in evaluating their automatic thoughts by helping them list the evidence for and against them. If necessary, do some research and find factual data that will help them challenge their maladaptive beliefs. This can be particularly useful when completing the "evidence against" section of the thought record.

Coping statements, or brief sentences that convey truth and optimism about the individual's ability to cope and the reality of the situation, are written in the last column and should be created with the client. Coping statements are the balanced, recovery-oriented statements that an individual creates at the end of the thought record after evaluating the full evidence for or against the automatic thoughts. For example, the coping statement might be "Even though it is difficult for me to take my medications because of the side effects, I realize that the benefits outweigh the consequences."

Another way to explain the process of thought change is to say that the individual is decreasing negative self-talk or creating a healthier internal dialogue. Problematic self-talk must be corrected for long-term change or relapse prevention to occur. Some examples of the kind of self-talk an individual with severe mental illness might engage in include "My disorder has ruined my life; I have nothing to live for now," "There is no way I can handle this," "I am such a failure," "Nobody will ever understand me," "Taking medication is not worth the side effects; I'd rather end up in the hospital," or "Nobody cares about me; I can't trust anyone." It is also good to help the individual replace extreme, catastrophizing words with more reasonable words. For example, ask if the situation is "challenging" as opposed to "unbearable," or "upsetting" rather than "devastating." Challenge the use of "always" by suggesting saying "often" or "many times" (Elliott & Smith, 2003). The chapters that follow provide sample thought change worksheets for each disorder.

Once clinicians become familiar with these fundamental tools and techniques, they will likely feel more confident and comfortable when helping clients who are experiencing psychiatric decompensation or a crisis state. Many of the strategies require only a beginner level of training and experience. Moderately challenging exercises can be conducted with more training and supervision. This chapter did not cover more advanced techniques, as these are tied to the specific disorders and covered in each chapter as relevant.

The next four chapters outline interventions that target specific psychiatric conditions. At times they include comments on how to tailor the fundamental tools and techniques to specific client populations. Also, interventions that have been proven effective for specific disorders are described. It may be necessary to go back and forth between the fundamentals chapter and the diagnosis-specific chapters when preparing interventions.

6

Schizophrenia and Schizoaffective Disorder

A 36-year-old man named Sam who is diagnosed with schizoaffective disorder was experiencing a significantly depressed mood and occasional homicidal ideation. He also reported hearing voices that others didn't hear, and he communicated in a disorganized manner much of the time. Sam had also maintained the delusional belief that his brother steals from him. Sam had run out of his medication several months ago and did not call to schedule an appointment with his psychiatrist. A combination of mood instability, drug use, and job and family frustration had caused Sam's negative feelings toward his brother, who lives with him and has bullied him for years, to intensify. He stated, "I'm just going to kill him; I can't take it anymore." He did not have a specific plan, but he needed help regaining control of his emotions through medication adherence, abstinence from drugs, and the development of new coping strategies.

*   *   *

Schizophrenia is a potentially disabling condition characterized by delusions, hallucinations, negative affect, limited interest, and interpersonal difficulty. Individuals diagnosed with schizoaffective disorder may present with similar symptoms, but they have also experienced significant mood episodes (depression or mania). These clients are more likely to have impaired emotional functioning in addition to the psychotic symptoms, while clients diagnosed with schizophrenia often have impaired cognitive functioning. These are likely the clients that most mental health professionals and lay people think of when they hear the term "serious mental illness."

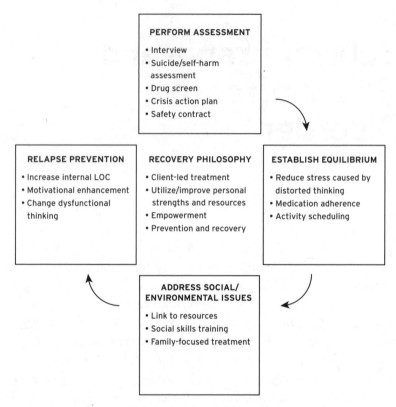

FIGURE 6.1   Schizophrenia and Schizoaffective Disorder

One of the best ways to understand the goal of treatment with psychotic clients is to consider the vulnerability-stress model of schizophrenia. According to Zubin and Spring (1977:109), the vulnerability model proposes that "each of us is endowed with a degree of vulnerability that under suitable circumstances will express itself in an episode of schizophrenic illness." In other words, many people have several psychological liabilities that make them susceptible to mental illness, such as schizophrenia, and given the right interpersonal and intrapersonal conditions, usually considerable and overwhelming stress, they will develop a particular disorder. Zubin and Spring explained the process further as follows:

> Trying to predict which individual will develop a disorder involves at least
> five factors: (a) the normatively perceived severity of the life event stressor,

(b) the individual's perception of the stressfulness of the load, (c) the capacities or general competence level of the individual in dealing with the stressful event, (d) the coping efforts exerted in dealing with the stressful situation, and (e) the vulnerability of the individual. (111)

Thus schizophrenia and other psychotic disorders often develop when a diminished capacity to manage stress is met with significant adverse events.

This process not only initiates the first psychotic break, it also causes relapse of psychotic episodes throughout the course of the illness (see appendix C, fig. 1). Zubin and Spring explain, "In the person vulnerable to schizophrenia, episodes of psychiatric disorder may often follow close on the heels of periods of acute stress and coping breakdown" (112). There are a number of psychological liabilities (see appendix C, fig. 2) that may cause an individual to have difficulty coping with stress (Preston, 2006). An assessment of current liabilities must be conducted throughout the treatment process so that the appropriate interventions are used. Vulnerability, or psychological liability, can be reduced through medication and psychosocial interventions, such as improving coping skills. It may also be helpful to explain the vulnerability-stress model to clients to increase their insight into the condition as well as the rationale for the various interventions. The figures provided in appendix C offer a simple yet sufficient way to explain the model.

PERFORM ASSESSMENT

Interview*

If clinicians are not already very familiar with the individual in crisis, then the assessment should be thorough enough to accurately assess psychotic and mood symptoms. This will help reduce mistakes in the treatment phase of the intervention. A good assessment will also improve communication among the treatment team and expedite the treatment process. The assessment interview will often reduce the client's anxiety, as the process gives the client the opportunity to discuss his or her concerns and stressors.

Building a strong therapeutic alliance with psychotic clients can be difficult at times, especially during an acute phase of the illness. Paranoia, misunderstanding about treatment goals and procedures, and irritability are among the reasons for this. Nonetheless, it is important to assess the specific symptoms being experienced, thoughts or events causing distress, and resources available to the client. Many times it will be necessary to consult with family members, friends, or other mental health professionals working with the client to get a full understanding of the current situation.

Some of the questions to ask regarding symptoms include:

- Are you having disturbing thoughts?
- Are you seeing things or hearing things that upset you?
- Do you feel that others are talking about you or want to hurt you in some way?
- Do you feel nervous, anxious, or worried? Did something happen recently that scared you or upset you?
- Has your mood been particularly low or high recently?

To assess recent social behavior and the status of the client's support system, clinicians could ask the following:

- What kinds of things have you been doing lately (work, visiting neighbors, watching TV, spending time alone)?
- How much time have you spent alone over the past few weeks? Is this normal?
- Do you talk or visit with family or friends?
- What have you done lately that was fun?
- Who do you enjoy spending time with? Have you seen that person recently?
- How are things where you are living? Is it stressful there? Do you have food, clothing, heat?

Many times these questions will lead to follow-up questions, and eventually clinicians will feel they have a solid picture of what is currently going on the client's life.

Suicide/Self-harm Assessment*

In one study patients diagnosed with schizophrenia who also had a history of self-harm had significantly greater symptoms of depression, greater suicidal thoughts, increased number of hospital admissions, and greater duration of illness compared to patients without a history of self-harm (Simms et al., 2007). All clients should be monitored for suicide or self-harm behavior, but those who match these characteristics may need to have specific goals related to suicide and self-harm included in their treatment plan. Clinicians should not hesitate to refer clients who are at high risk for suicide to inpatient care if community-based services are having minimal success with the stabilization process.

Drug Screen*

Issues such as suspiciousness or paranoia may need to be addressed with psychotic clients before and during the drug screen. Being very specific about the details of the procedure and confidentiality might reduce anxiety. Follow the process outlined in chapter 5.

Crisis Action Plan*

An important issue to address with psychotic clients is harm reduction. For instance, if clients have a history of violence toward themselves or others, it will be necessary to ensure that their environment is as safe as it can be. Weapons or potentially dangerous objects should be removed. Staff should be deliberate in creating safety procedures for home visits, group sessions, office visits, and so forth. If substance abuse is an issue, an effort should be made to prevent access to substances and to monitor drug-seeking behavior. Furthermore, since many psychotic clients are at high risk for suicide, a specific plan should be established in case of a psychiatric emergency (i.e., suicidal thoughts, psychotic disturbance, and intense hopelessness). The client should be provided with crisis hotline numbers and a list of coping strategies. This information should be written in clear language on the Crisis Action Plan (appendix A). Individuals who have borderline intellectual functioning or mental retardation may need simplified instructions, reminders posted around the home, and frequent review of the plan.

Contracts*

Contracts with this client population could involve committing to refrain from drug or alcohol use, taking medications as prescribed, staying away from particular people or places, and talking to someone when experiencing strong emotions. For those who become paranoid around signing their name, a verbal commitment will suffice. The key is to provide accountability and positive reinforcement by giving them a challenge, or a goal, and to reward them with praise when they are successful.

.   .   .

Sam was clearly experiencing distress when his case manager (CM) came to see him at his home. He was reluctant to talk to the CM because he was agitated and did not want to discuss how he was feeling. The CM explained to Sam that she was worried because he looked tired and he was showing the same symptoms that he had before his most recent hospitalization. Rather than threatening Sam with calling emergency services to have him prescreened if he did not cooperate, the CM sat with him for a while and talked with him about things he typically enjoys talking about. Eventually Sam began to share that he had not been sleeping and had begun hearing voices again. He claimed the voices told him he was a bad person and he was worthless, and this caused him to get angry and to lose sleep. The CM suspected that Sam might be using marijuana again because his symptoms of hallucinatory behavior, irritability, and isolation were consistent with previous relapses. Sam was asked if he had been using alcohol or drugs. He admitted he has been using marijuana nearly every day to keep from going "crazy." Later it was determined that he was self-medicating to avoid experiencing a manic episode. Sam was asked if he had stopped taking his medication, and he stated that he ran out about four months ago. The CM asked Sam if he had experienced thoughts of hurting himself; Sam said, "No, but I have thought about punching my brother in the face." The CM knew that Sam did not have a history of self-harm or violence toward others, but his level of irritability caused some concern.

Sam was escorted to the mental health center, where he met with his psychiatrist. The CM explained that Sam was showing signs of decompensation and had not been taking his medication. The psychiatrist and CM talked with Sam about how the marijuana use can be connected to his current symptoms. Sam explained that he uses the marijuana to prevent feeling manic. The doctor told him that taking the medication and finding ways to reduce stress will also prevent mania, and if he is going to stay out of the hospital he will need to begin taking his medication regularly again. Sam verbally contracted to stop using marijuana and to begin taking his medication again. He also agreed to try to limit interactions with his brother. The CM took Sam back to his home

and assisted him in filling out his crisis action plan. They added the informa-
tion that had already been discussed regarding Sam's triggers, symptoms, and
recovery strategies and made sure he had appropriate phone numbers in case
his symptoms worsened. The case manager told Sam she would meet with him
again the following day.

ESTABLISH EQUILIBRIUM

Reduce Distress Caused by Distorted Thinking***

Strategies for tolerating hallucinations can be taught to this client population. For example, Kingdon and Turkington (2005) suggested that clients can use the following methods for reducing distress caused by hearing
voices:

- Turn on the radio or TV (or off if the voices seem to be coming from it) or
  listen to music with headphones.
- Talk to a friend, go for a walk, be active.
- Read a newspaper, book, or magazine.
- Develop a relationship with the voices and ask why they are saying what
  they say, or challenge them when they say bad things.
- Understand that voices cannot make you do anything.

Kingdon and Turkington also suggest the following methods for reducing stress caused by ideas of reference and thought broadcasting:

- Keep a diary of incidences when the radio, TV, newspaper, or a stranger
  seems to be referring to you or when you feel others know what you are
  thinking.
- Discuss the diary with someone (e.g., family, mental health worker).
- Contemplate, with a supportive person, why they would be referring to you
  or know your thoughts.

It is not uncommon for clients who are experiencing psychotic symptoms to become angry. This could be due to confusion, frustration, paranoia, or other things. It is likely that the client is experiencing distortions
in thinking, and distress can be lessened if these thoughts are identified and
challenged. McKay and Rogers (2000) provide a list of anger distortions
and ways to counter the distortions. Some of these are as follows:

- Magnifying/exaggeration—be realistically negative; use accurate language; look at the whole picture.
- Overgeneralization—avoid general terms and use specific ones; look for exceptions to the rule.
- Misattribution—check out your assumptions about other people's motives; consider alternative explanations.

Medication Adherence*

Issues related to medication adherence among psychotic clients may include paranoia surrounding the medication or prescribing physician, negative side-effects, and confusion about which medications to take and at what times. It is often necessary to fill a pillbox for these clients on a weekly basis, and during an acute period of their illness it may be helpful to monitor medication adherence daily. It may also be necessary to find a mental health worker or family member whom the client trusts to facilitate conversations around medication adherence.

Activity Scheduling*

This is not the time to refer clients to clubhouse programs or support groups as these can overstimulate and the client may respond negatively, thus sabotaging future opportunities. Instead, start by increasing time spent outside of the client's room or home and work on engagement with people and activities the client likes, then build up to more intense social activities as the client stabilizes. Follow the recommendations for increasing activity discussed in chapter 5.

●   ●   ●

The case manager asked Sam if he had taken his medication the previous evening and he said he had. He also stated that he did not use marijuana. Sam continued to demonstrate irritability and overall dysphoria (unpleasant mood), but he said the voices hadn't been bothering him much today. The CM explained to Sam there are many different ways to improve his mood and that over the next few days she would be helping him learn and practice some of these strategies to try to prevent hospitalization. The CM began by describing the various coping skills and by having Sam select the ones he was willing to try. Sam decided to begin taking walks when he felt upset and to listen to relaxing music while at home.

The CM spent the rest of the visit talking with Sam about his reasons for stopping his medication a few months ago. Sam said he did not feel that it worked and that he was concerned about gaining weight. The CM responded empathically and reviewed with Sam the various negative and positive aspects of taking the medication, supportively correcting false information along the way. For instance, she informed Sam that she could see a significant difference in his mood and behavior when he stopped taking his medication and that the weight gain will eventually stop. Sam agreed that the benefits outweighed the costs because he does not want to become homeless or end up in the hospital.

One of the reasons Sam began to experience an increase in agitation and paranoid thoughts toward his brother was that he had become very isolated. To integrate Sam back into the community so that he could begin to interact with others and feel socially connected, the CM helped Sam create an activity schedule. Sam decided to start by spending more time outside on his porch and by talking with some of his neighbors more. His activity progressed to a point where he was going fishing at a pier, where he new several people. Sam was held accountable for engaging in his scheduled activities during the following meetings. His use of coping skills, medication adherence, and activity was reinforced through encouragement from the CM and the reduction in symptom severity.

ADDRESS SOCIAL AND ENVIRONMENTAL ISSUES

General Tips*

This might include ensuring the client has necessary food, shelter, bedding, and heating or cooling. Additionally, issues related to darkness or noise can often be easily resolved for clients who experience psychosis or discomfort in specific situations. Follow the general tips for addressing potential environmental stressors described earlier.

Social Skills Training*

• *Assertiveness.* Assertiveness training can be used to reduce aggressive behavior often found among individuals with psychotic disorders. For many clients with psychosis, cognitive or intellectual deficits contribute to aggressive behavior. Modeling appropriate assertive communication can help them to have their needs met without annoying or offending others. It can also help them to be active participants in the planning of their treatment. Follow the instructions for assertiveness training provided in chapter 5.

• *Communication.* Model good communication skills (e.g., effective listening, clear messages) and help the client recognize times and ways that he or she could communicate (both verbally and nonverbally) more effectively. For instance, if the client has a tendency to demand assistance from family members, mental health professionals, or others, demonstrate how to respectfully ask for assistance so that one's needs are more likely to be met.

• *Self-monitoring.* This refers to the client's ability to recognize when a behavior is abnormal or disruptive as well as the ability to make necessary adjustments. Help individuals become more competent in evaluating their behavior by taking advantage of opportunities to comment on both prosocial and antisocial behaviors. For instance, if a female client is annoying those around her by singing loudly while listening to headphones, help her to realize how others are experiencing her, so she is able to catch herself and make the proper adjustment.

Family-Focused Treatment**

Family-focused treatment aims to provide the client with a stable and stress-free environment by improving communication (e.g., reducing verbal hostility) between client and family and by regulating expressed emotion (e.g., decreasing emotional overinvolvement) among family members. These issues are addressed through a combination of education, communication enhancement training, and problem-solving skills training. The treatment strategies are outlined by Miklowitz (2002) as follows.

ASSESSMENT

• How does the family communicate (e.g., do they listen attentively and non-judgmentally or tune out and criticize)?
• Are various opinions treated fairly, or does one person dominate?
• Do problems ever get solved, or do family members refuse to agree?
• What is the emotional nature of conversations—are family members highly charged or very passive and withdrawn?

EDUCATION

- Describe the typical symptoms of schizophrenia (e.g., visual, auditory, or tactile hallucinations; disorganized speech or behavior; lack of interest in or ability to feel pleasure from activities; limited range of emotional expression; paranoid thoughts) or schizoaffective disorder (symptoms of schizophrenia and depressive and/or manic symptoms).
- Assist the client and family in identifying precipitants to psychotic and mood episodes and explain that the client may be particularly vulnerable to stress based on his or her biological makeup.
- Explain how medication and counseling can make the client less likely to have a negative response to stress through regulating internal and external vulnerabilities. Also, explain the role of the family in reducing stress and responding to relapse.

COMMUNICATION ENHANCEMENT

- Teach listening skills (McKay, Fanning, & Paleg, 1994). Examples of bad listening include mind reading (making assumptions), sparring (listening only to disagree and build ammunition to argue a position), judging (no longer listening after judging the person as an idiot, closed-minded, and so forth). Ways to improve listening include using good body language such as eye contact and facing the person, paraphrasing, and clarifying.
- Teach general communication skills (McKay, Fanning, & Paleg, 1994). These include using clear and whole messages, avoiding threats, avoiding judgmental language, and avoiding exaggeration (e.g., always, never). Careful (versus reckless) criticism and confrontation, for example, means sandwiching a criticism or complaint between two compliments, or sandwiching a negative between two positives. For example, "Hey Robert, I know you are not feeling well right now and you are trying hard to relax, but I really need you to stop yelling—can you go for a walk or something? I appreciate you helping me out" versus "Robert, shut up, you are making me crazy."

PROBLEM-SOLVING SKILLS

- Be flexible, be persistent (don't easily give up on negotiation), separate feelings from the issue, do not get caught in the blame game (McKay, Fanning, & Paleg, 1994).

- Use role playing and discussion about real or hypothetical scenarios to help guide the family through problem-solving steps: define the problem, generate possible solutions, assess pros and cons of each solution, choose the best solution, and carry out the plan (Miklowitz, 2002).

      •   •   •

Since Sam relies on his brother for financial support and housing, it was important to try to make their relationship more stable and healthy. With Sam's consent, the CM asked the brother to meet with her and Sam during her next two visits. During the first meeting the CM provided brief education about Sam's mental illness and explained to the brother that there are things he can do to avoid exacerbating Sam's symptoms. She explained that when people with illness similar to Sam's are around people with a high level of negative emotional expression, they have difficulty staying emotionally and mentally stable and their symptoms worsen. The brother, who is quite loud and animated, explained that he tries to stay calm around Sam but his personality gets in the way. During the second joint meeting, the CM reviewed with Sam and his brother various ways they can begin to improve their interactions. She taught them how to communicate and problem solve effectively. She also talked with the brother about his tendency to be critical of Sam and to push him to do things like work, go out on the weekends, and complete chores around the house when he cannot really tolerate this level of activity. The brother reluctantly agreed to place fewer demands on Sam until he is more stable and to work on being more supportive.

Another issue that makes Sam vulnerable to stress is his poor social skills. Sam is used to giving into other people's wishes because he has relied on others ever since becoming ill. He has lost his ability to assert his opinion and to ask for assistance when he needs help. Also, he has become increasingly uncomfortable in social situations and disorganized in his speech and appearance because of his isolative behavior. As Sam was encouraged to become more socially involved, his CM also reminded him about his personal rights and encouraged him to use assertive versus aggressive behavior. She also educated him about effective communication and ways to set up appropriate boundaries. Sam was assisted in practicing self-monitoring by asking him how he thinks others might be perceiving him when he does not use proper hygiene or engages in antisocial or strange behavior. Eventually Sam became better able to read social cues and to adjust his behavior appropriately. This reduced stress by increasing positive social interaction with others.

RELAPSE PREVENTION

Increase Internal Locus of Control*

For the individual who has been institutionalized, this empowerment intervention might be necessary but challenging. Be patient, go at a steady pace, and continuously try to increase the client's perception of personal control. This fundamental intervention is similar for all conditions.

Motivation Enhancement*

Use the various motivational interviewing strategies discussed earlier to improve treatment participation and to encourage the continuation of recovery-promoting behavior after treatment. These strategies can be used to help the client overcome barriers to a variety of changes that need to be made, such as medication adherence, ceasing drug use, and engaging in social activity.

Change Dysfunctional Thinking**

When working with the psychotic client, it is common to discover cognitive errors or problematic thinking. The thought change worksheet at the end of this chapter can be used to address a number of these issues. The targeted thoughts often revolve around treatment adherence. Sometimes the targeted thoughts will be related to depression and feelings of worthlessness or hopelessness. At other times it is necessary to address faulty beliefs about others, such as family and treatment providers. Clients can also benefit from the thought change worksheet because it can help to facilitate reality testing and to challenge destructive delusional systems. Consider these ideas while following the general instructions for using the thought change worksheet.

Cognitive therapy has been found to be effective in decreasing the strength and thus the negative consequences of delusions (Kingdon & Turkington, 2005; Chadwick, Birchwood, Trower, 1996). Although, cognitive therapy for psychosis is most often conducted over a period of several

TABLE 6.1

DELUSION	ANTECEDENT	BELIEF	CONSEQUENCE
Mind reading	During a conversation the doctor finishes a sentence for the person.	She read my mind; people know what I am thinking.	Feels exposed, isolates, avoids interaction with staff.
Paranoid	Therapist discusses information learned by reading the chart.	This is some kind of conspiracy; how did you get that information?	Fearful, confused, becomes combative.
Reference	Person begins to think critical judge on popular TV show is chastising him.	I haven't done anything wrong; why am I in trouble? They always blame me.	Shameful, angry, goes away from TV upset.
Somatic	Person develops an itchy rash.	I'm infested with bugs.	Feels horror, scratches vigorously.
Grandiose	Person is randomly selected to be part of new peer-support class at a day treatment center.	They know I am intelligent; I'm smarter than anyone here.	Excited, feels urgency to share new evidence of superiority; peers are annoyed.

weeks and by highly trained clinicians, an understanding of the cognitive model of delusions as well as the ability to use a simple tool for challenging delusions can be of great benefit to mental health professionals of all levels who regularly work with psychotic clients. The two main goals of using cognitive therapy to address delusions are to weaken the delusions and to weaken the associated negative evaluative thoughts (Chadwick, Birchwood, Trower, 1996). Although problematic delusional thinking and associated hallucinations may not be fully resolved during the acute care intervention, addressing these issues even briefly could go a long way in establishing stability. It should be noted, however, that a healthy alliance between the clinician and client is required for this mode of treatment to be successful.

The first step is to understand the ABC model, on which cognitive therapy is based. The A stands for the activating event or trigger. B stands for beliefs and includes images, thoughts, and attitudes the individual experiences following the event. Lastly, C represents the consequences or positive and negative effects of the triggered images, thoughts, or beliefs. Although simplistic, this model helps us conceptualize how events are connected to behaviors through cognitive processes. The ABC model can be applied to delusions in a way similar to that shown in table 6.1.

Kingdon & Turkington (2005) provide the following tips for successfully challenging or weakening delusions:

- Focus on facilitating exploration of alternatives and avoid confrontation.
- Use the prompts "Any other possible explanations for what happened?"; "What about...?"; "Do you think possibly...?"
- Bring in people the client respects and will listen to. Bring them in either physically or simply by saying, "What does _____ think about that idea?" or "Why do you think your sister thinks that?"

* * *

Sam is proud of the fact that he is able to stop using marijuana when he feels like it and uses this to defend using it. Over the past two weeks he has reported abstinence from drug or alcohol use, but he has a history of going back to smoking and stopping his medication when he begins to feel significant distress. To prevent relapse, Sam will have to become more serious about his recovery and stay committed to his treatment program. Sam's CM used motivational interviewing strategies during the next several visits to help Sam stay focused on his recovery. She used Sam's goal of living independently and being healthy enough to work again to keep him motivated to engage in all the stress-reducing activities he has learned. She also helped Sam to develop a greater sense of control over his life by intentionally pointing out the direct cause-and-effect relationship between Sam's behavior and his mood as well as his interactions with others and their response. This allowed Sam to see that although many things are out of his control, including various biological and situational vulnerabilities, he is still able to work toward recovery, and his effort most certainly matters.

When Sam's emotional and cognitive functioning had improved to a point where he could process some of the thoughts that are contributing to his distress, the CM introduced him to the thought change worksheet. She explained to Sam that sometimes people have thoughts that are based on faulty assumptions or incorrect data, and that it is important to be able to identify when this problem is occurring and to correct it. She used several hypothetical examples

TABLE 6.2 Thought Change Worksheet—Example (Sam)

SITUATION	RESPONSE	AUTOMATIC THOUGHTS	EVIDENCE THAT SUPPORTS THE TROUBLE THOUGHT	EVIDENCE THAT DOES NOT SUPPORT THE TROUBLE THOUGHT	ALTERNATIVE / BALANCED THOUGHTS
Describe what is (was) going on at the time you experience(d) distress. Who? What? When? Where?	a. What do (did) you feel? b. Use specific emotion words like angry, sad, helpless, scared, hurt, hopeless, disappointed.	a. What was going through your mind just before you started to feel this way? Any Images? b. Circle the trouble thought (the one most connected to the distress).	List the facts that suggest the trouble thought is true.	List the facts that suggest the trouble thought is not true.	a. Write an alternative or balanced thought considering the facts. b. Rate how much you believe in the alternative or balanced thought (0–10).
It is the morning on Monday and I can't find my pack of cigarettes. My brother is at work and I've been inside all day.	Angry Frustrated Anxious	I'm going to kill my brother for taking my cigarettes. My brother is always stealing from me. I hate living with my brother. I just can't trust anyone. Everyone steals from me.	My brother is mean to me a lot and picks on me. A lot of my stuff ends of missing.	I've never seen my brother actually take something of mine. Sometimes I find the things I've lost in my room. My brother doesn't smoke.	My brother may not have stolen my cigarettes. I just don't know how things go missing. (9)

to show Sam how the thought change worksheet helps to identify problematic thoughts and to challenge the accuracy of the thoughts. When Sam felt confident that he understood the process, the CM began to help him challenge the delusional thought that his brother steals from him. Each time Sam would tell the CM that something was stolen, she would use the worksheet to challenge this belief, and eventually Sam began to initiate the process on his own. After a few months of using the thought change worksheet, Sam was less likely to accuse his brother of stealing, and his overall experience of paranoia decreased.

7

Major Depression and Bipolar Disorder

Mary, a 44-year-old single woman diagnosed with bipolar disorder, was depressed and reported she had experienced suicidal ideation over the past few days. She was tearful, irritable, anxious, and complaining of "feeling bad all the time." She repeated several times, "I'm just so stupid" and "I can't do anything right." Mary has been struggling with alcohol addiction for several years and recently relapsed after two years of sobriety. Also, her boyfriend left her nearly three months ago, which was very difficult for her. She has burned nearly all of her bridges with family and friends over the past several years because of her behavior while intoxicated, so her current support system is very limited and primarily consists of her AA group and case manager. She has difficulty gathering the courage and energy to get out of her home, and she sleeps most of the day. Mary did not want to go to the hospital but needed assistance in achieving an increased level of self-control and psychiatric stability.

· · ·

Bipolar disorder typically involves a history of manic or hypomanic episodes (e.g., elevated, expansive, or irritable mood; inflated self-esteem; decreased need for sleep; pressured speech; excessive thrill seeking) and one or more major depressive episodes. Symptom presentations can vary, but the onset of mania is often marked by a mood that has either become exceedingly euphoric or extremely irritable. Medication is usually required to treat clients who experience a manic episode, while a combination of

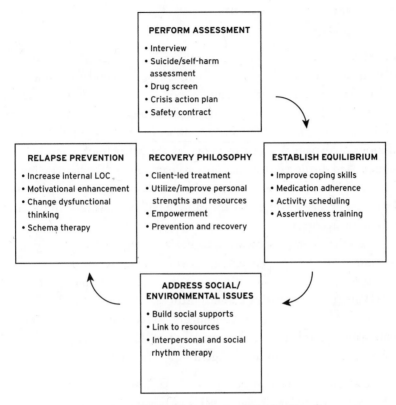

FIGURE 7.1 Major Depression and Bipolar Disorder

medication and psychosocial intervention is best for those experiencing a depressive episode.

Major depressive disorder is one of the most commonly diagnosed psychiatric illnesses. The symptom presentation can vary as some clients have more somatic, or physical, complaints while others may have poor social functioning or behavioral problems. Some of the most common symptoms associated with major depression include feelings of guilt, fatigue, poor concentration, irritable mood and agitation, suicidal thoughts and thoughts of death, appetite changes, sleep disturbance, low self-esteem and self-critical thinking, decreased pleasure, and withdrawal and avoidance.

PERFORM ASSESSMENT

Interview*

If the clinician is not already very familiar with the individual in crisis, the assessment should be thorough enough to ensure an understanding of the specific characteristics of the client's symptoms, which will help to reduce mistakes in selecting, implementing, and communicating about the interventions. Many different factors can influence one's mood: activity level, relationship dynamics, access to resources, the behavior of others, self-perception, and disrupted sleep patterns, to name a few. The better clinicians are able to identify the factors that are currently causing an exacerbation of depressive or manic symptoms, the easier it will be to work with the client to facilitate recovery.

When the client presents with mania, it is important to perform a risk assessment that addresses potential for violence; degree of financial harm; risky sexual behavior-exploitation; spread of communicable diseases such as HIV, herpes, or hepatitis C; and history of running away. With either condition it is important to continually assess whether the individual's acute symptomatology includes suicidal or self-harm behavior.

Some of the questions to ask regarding symptoms include:

- Has your mood been particularly low or high recently?
- Do you feel as though your thoughts are racing?
- Are you having difficulty concentrating?
- Do you feel nervous, anxious, or worried?
- Did something happen recently that scared you or upset you?
- Has your energy level changed?
- What are some of your current thoughts and feelings?
- What has your sleep been like?

Use the list of questions in the same section of chapter 6 to assess recent social behavior and the status of the client's support system for a complete understanding of what is currently going on in the client's life.

Suicide/Self-harm Assessment*

It is imperative that clinicians assess suicidality in mood-disordered individuals experiencing a crisis. Some of the risk factors for suicide among clients with bipolar disorder include previous suicide attempts or violent acts, previous severe and frequently recurring depression, substance-use comorbidity, current depression or dysphoric-agitated states, hopelessness, current stressors (e.g., loss, separation, medical illness, financial crisis), impulsivity, and ready access to firearms or toxins (Tondo, Isacsson, & Baldessarini, 2003; Fagiolini et al., 2004). Salient risk factors for suicide among depressed clients include prior suicide attempts, a desire to die, hopelessness, psychotic features, guilt, comorbid substance use, significant physical illness, personality disorder, permanent stressors (e.g., dysfunctional marriage, physical handicap), mixed-state depression/agitation, family history of suicide, lack of social support, and a recent adverse life situation (Gonda et al., 2007).

It is not uncommon for suicide risk to increase as a person's depression begins to weaken (Joiner, 2005). If the individual has already committed to a plan of action, the increased energy and mental clarity may be what is necessary to complete the act. Therefore the client's mood cannot be the only target of suicide assessment. Issues that increase suicide risk should be assessed and addressed throughout the intervention.

Drug Screen*

Many mood-disordered clients engage in substance abuse. Not only does this cause depression to worsen, as well as create other difficulties, it can also increase risk for suicide. Follow the recommendations for assessing substance use described in the fundamental tools and techniques chapter and attempt to reduce this risk factor. Provide referrals for substance abuse treatment if necessary.

Crisis Action Plan*

As mentioned previously, an important issue to address with clients experiencing bipolar illness is harm reduction during manic episodes. For instance, if the client has a history of spending sprees, it is important to have a plan regarding who will control bank and credit cards. Likewise, if substance abuse is an issue during manic or depressive episodes, an effort should be made to prevent access to substances and to monitor drug-seeking behavior. Furthermore, since depressed and bipolar clients are at high risk for suicide, a specific plan should be established in case of a psychiatric emergency. As always, the client should be provided with crisis hotline numbers and a list of coping strategies. A severely depressed individual will likely need significant help with generating ideas when completing the crisis action plan.

Contracts*

Understand that a client's signature or agreement is no guarantee that he or she will not engage in self-harm behavior; therefore, continued vigilance around this issue is necessary. Also, remember that even if a depressed client with a recent history of suicidal ideation appears to be feeling better, the potential for completed suicide may not be any less. Sometimes those with severe depression have committed to end their life and are just waiting for the energy to complete their plan. Follow the recommendations for using contracts described in chapter 5.

                    •   •   •

Mary was assessed at the community mental health center by the assertive community treatment team coordinator. Mary had been receiving case management and other services through the ACT team for nearly a year, but her contact with them had been minimal over the past two months because she had successfully avoided them. When the clinician asked Mary where she had been and how she had been doing over the past several weeks, it became evident that Mary had experienced a manic episode. Mary explained that her relationship with her boyfriend was chaotic, she was having problems with coworkers at her part-time job, and she was having difficulty sleeping. The stress became overwhelming, and Mary began to experience intense irritability, racing thoughts, and increased goal-driven and risk-taking behavior. During this episode Mary had stopped taking her medication and did not feel the need to go to medical appointments. She also stated that she began using alcohol again.

Mary had recently switched to the depressed phase of her illness and she was feeling shameful about her relapse, sad about losing her boyfriend, and hopeless because she had worked hard toward recovery over the past two years. The clinician was aware that Mary has a history of at least two suicide attempts by way of medication overdose and that she used to cut her arms when she was a teenager. So the clinician asked if Mary had recently thought about hurting herself or ending her life, and Mary reported that she had thought about overdosing a couple of times because her bottles were full since she had not taken the medication for several weeks. She then told the ACT coordinator that she didn't want to die and probably would not do anything to hurt herself; she just didn't know what to do right now.

The clinician reviewed with Mary some of the coping strategies that had been helpful in the past and taught her some new ones. She helped Mary create a list of activities she could use and add to her crisis action plan, and made sure she had the number of the mental health center's crisis hotline. Additionally, Mary agreed to ask her roommate to hold onto her pill bottles after she filled her weekly pill box. The clinician contacted the team psychiatrist and explained the situation; he approved of having Mary begin taking her medication as previously prescribed. The clinician had Mary write and sign a contract to not harm herself or use alcohol over the next twenty-four hours and then scheduled a time to meet with her the following day.

ESTABLISH EQUILIBRIUM

Improving Coping Skills*

For both manic and depressed clients, the recommended coping strategies will often require the support of others. Also, it is important to work on increasing motivation and teaching coping skills simultaneously with these individuals. Common coping strategies during a depressive episode include distraction strategies, self-soothing, and increasing contact with supportive others. For those experiencing a manic episode, coping often involves managing impulsive behavior by reducing access to things like credit cards and alcohol or drugs. Avoiding stimulants, engaging in physical activity, and relaxation techniques might also be used. Follow the recommendations for improving the client's ability to manage distress described in chapter 5.

Medication Adherence*

Medication adherence can be particularly difficult when a client is manic and experiencing euphoria. The individual will likely argue that he or she feels well and does not see the need for medicine. In these cases it can be helpful to solicit assistance from trusted family or mental health professionals in the effort to persuade the client to take medication regularly. Follow the recommendations for improving medication adherence outlined chapter 5.

Activity Scheduling*

Increasing social and physical activity can be an essential yet difficult task for individuals experiencing moderate to severe depression. Motivation enhancement strategies will likely need to be used while developing an activity schedule. Furthermore, peer support can be helpful for the client in the effort to find things to do and to follow through with participation. It is important to guard against stimulus overload by offering or suggesting activities that range in level of participation and physical and emotional exertion. This will prevent failed attempts at increasing activity, which could result in a diminished level of self-esteem and self-efficacy. The general recommendations for increasing activity discussed in chapter 5 should also be followed.

Assertiveness Training*

This activity can help empower depressed clients to break patterns of victimization and to decrease feelings of hopelessness. This might be a significant challenge for individuals who have a high level of perceived helplessness and low levels of self-esteem and self-efficacy. Assistance with this strategy is provided in chapter 5.

•   •   •

The ACT team staff met with Mary daily and reviewed with her the various coping skills. Mary began using deep breathing and relaxation as well as self-soothing strategies when she became anxious or irritable. She and a staff member spent one session creating an activity schedule so that she could begin to get out of her home and do some of the things she enjoys. The first goal was to have her maintain good hygiene each day and clean her room each morning. She gradually progressed to taking walks outside her apartment twice a day and cooking meals, and these activities began to significantly improve her mood.

She adhered to her medication schedule with very little prompting, but ACT staff continued to ask her about this during each visit.

One of the primary stressors affecting Mary was her inability to have her needs met. This occurred at her part-time job and in interpersonal relationships. Mary's employment was in jeopardy because she had been missing days to avoid coworkers who make condescending remarks and treat her unfairly. She claimed she often feels helpless and is reluctant to tell her supervisor of the situation because she doesn't know how to approach him and is concerned that he will not be supportive. To help address this issue, Mary was taught assertiveness skills such as effective communication, expressing her needs, setting clear boundaries, and voicing her opinion through role-playing. She became increasingly aware of her rights and more confident in her ability to defend them after a few sessions. The assertiveness training also helped her to say no to peers who offered her alcohol and to avoid ending up in various locations that might trigger her desire to use alcohol.

ADDRESS SOCIAL AND ENVIRONMENTAL ISSUES

General Tips*

For the depressed client, increasing positive social contact and limiting contact with those who often contribute to stress are important. Sometimes it is possible to combine strategies, such as signing the client up for a "meals-on-wheels" or similar program so that he or she will receive daily contact and good nutrition. Something that might be overlooked at times is the use of social networking, online support groups, and other Internet-based opportunities to increase socialization or explore interests. Clinicians might provide a quick tutorial for computer owners who are feeling lonely, bored, or hopeless. Also, follow the general recommendations for addressing social and environmental issues described in chapter 5.

Interpersonal and Social Rhythm Therapy (IPSRT)**

Interpersonal therapy is a technique that involves helping the client focus on a specific and current problem area, and targeting the issue with appropriate strategies (Swartz, Markowitz, & Frank, 2002). According to Swartz and colleagues, there are four general interpersonal problem areas: grief (e.g., loss of loved one), role disputes (e.g., repeated arguments with spouse about responsibilities), interpersonal role transitions (e.g., children moving away, job loss/change, moving), and interpersonal deficits (history of unsuccessful relationships—no specific stressor). They offer the following suggestions for intervention in each problem area.

GRIEF

- Talk with the client about the lost person(s) and the meaning of their relationship.
- Encourage the expression of emotion while meeting with the client (i.e., combat tendency to suppress).
- Carefully help the client to recognize distorted thoughts, memories, or attributions and provide healthy alternatives.
- Help the client to accept the idea that changes may need to be made, and facilitate the effort to reengage in activities and other relationships.

INTERPERSONAL ROLE DISPUTE

- Identify the persons involved in the dispute and the exact nature of the conflict.
- Develop a plan for change (explore realistic and safe options; desired outcome is resolution of the conflict or ending the relationship; might need to include other person).
- Assist the client in improving communication patterns and changing expectations (role-play).

ROLE TRANSITION

- Help the client to evaluate characteristics of new role (e.g., mother, widow, unemployed) and the ways in which it differs from the old role, and to develop a balanced view of these roles.
- Help the client to effectively mourn the loss of the old role while facilitating necessary skill development for the new role.

INTERPERSONAL DEFICITS

- Educate the client about the relationship between mood symptoms and difficulties in social functioning (i.e., the reciprocal relationship).

- Teach social skills such as assertiveness, effective communication, appropriate boundaries, and identifying dangerous situations.

Regulating social rhythms (sleep patterns, meal times, exercise routines, social activity) has also been shown to decrease risk for new mood episodes, especially mania, among individuals with bipolar disorder (Swartz, Markowitz, & Frank, 2002). Therefore it is important to assist the client in evaluating sleep-wake patterns and to help determine ways to improve quality and consistency in these patterns. Ways to improve sleep include making the bedroom environment comfortable (cool, quiet, dark), exercising in the afternoon, taking a relaxing bath or shower before going to bed, establishing a regular pattern of sleep, avoiding daytime naps, and avoiding eating heavy foods and drinking caffeinated beverages before bedtime (Van Brunt & Lichstein, 2000). It is also important for clients to take their medications at a consistent time because many of them have sedating or stimulating effects that influence sleep.

Clinicians can also help the client establish a set schedule for eating. This may be more difficult for those who have a variable work schedule or large families. Another issue that may need to be addressed is the client's work schedule. If someone is working too much or even inconsistently, he or she may be vulnerable to mood episodes. The key is to establish external stability so that the client's internal, physiological rhythms are also stable. With medication and stable social rhythms, the client should begin to feel more in control of the symptoms. Clients should be encouraged to assess the status of their social rhythms each week to determine whether there are disruptions that need to be addressed. Therapists, case managers, or family members can assist with this.

•   •   •

Mary shares a small apartment with another woman who has a severe mental illness at a supportive living complex run by the community mental health agency. Although they get along fairly well and her roommate is typically supportive, Mary is having difficulty sharing the small space. Additionally, her roommate has a history of substance use and recently began dating a man who abuses alcohol. He has been bringing alcohol to the apartment for Mary, and they have been drinking together since her relapse. One of the ACT team case managers scheduled a meeting with the residential program director and Mary to address the issue. The roommate's boyfriend was prevented from coming to the apartment, and eventually Mary was moved to a single-occupancy apartment. She agreed to return to the AA meetings she had previously been attending at least three times a week to receive support in her effort to battle the negative influences around her.

Mary had also run out of food because she had been spending her money on alcohol over the past few weeks. She was taken to the Salvation Army to get a box of food as well as a clothing voucher so she could get a new pair of pants and shirt for her return to work. ACT staff encouraged her to buy food as soon as she received her next check so that she was less tempted to spend her money on something else.

Mary has experienced multiple interpersonal problems over the past year. Her behavior has caused her family to stop initiating interaction with her, and she has been unable to establish healthy dating relationships. She is also having trouble getting along with coworkers. ACT team workers began helping Mary to improve her interpersonal deficits by providing education about how her behavior affects others and by reinforcing positive social interactions with staff through encouragement and praise. Staff also continued to work with her on her assertiveness and problem-solving skills so that she will be less susceptible to peer influence and more effective in her social interactions.

The ACT team assisted Mary in her effort to establish equilibrium and improve her daily social functioning by helping her regulate her social rhythms. To establish a structured daily schedule, the staff had Mary choose a specific time at night to go to sleep as well as a nighttime routine that will help her relax and sleep well. She also chose specific meal times and was encouraged to avoid skipping meals. She was discouraged from taking naps during the day and encouraged to follow her activity schedule.

RELAPSE PREVENTION

Increase Internal Locus of Control*

Depressed clients often attribute problems in their life to personal factors (low self-esteem), yet they believe the ability to make changes lies in external factors (low self-efficacy). These clients will feel empowered as they begin to share some of the responsibility for their negative circumstances with the various related external forces and will begin to play an active role in their recovery as the control they have over how they respond to their circumstances is highlighted.

Motivation Enhancement*

A motivational interviewing approach has been suggested as a way to increase the level of engagement in the treatment process for clients with bipolar disorder (Otto & Reilly-Harrington, 2002) and major depression (Zuckoff, Swartz, & Grote, 2008). Follow the recommendations for improving motivation outlined in chapter 5. Significant prompting might be necessary to assist the depressed client with identifying goals and imagining positive changes.

Change Dysfunctional Thinking**

When working with clients diagnosed with bipolar disorder, the targeted thoughts usually revolve around treatment adherence. These clients can also benefit from the thought change worksheet as they are recovering from a manic phase because it can help facilitate reality testing and challenge residual grandiosity or other symptoms. At times thoughts related to being diagnosed with bipolar disorder and having to adjust to various new limitations will be targeted.

Severely depressed clients can use this technique to challenge pessimism about the future as well as excessive negativity regarding their abilities, behaviors, looks, and other things that contribute to their distress. It can be difficult for these clients to come up with healthy alternatives to their dysfunctional thoughts, so clinicians must be prepared to assist them with this task. Some examples of the kind of self-talk a client with a mood disorder might engage in include "Bipolar/depression has ruined my life; I have nothing to live for now," "There is no way I can handle this," "I am such a failure," "Nobody will ever understand me," "If I take medication I will be a zombie and my life will be pointless," and "It is better to be manic than depressed."

Schema Therapy***

Schemas are lifelong characterological themes that comprise memories, emotions, cognitions, and sensations regarding oneself and one's relationships with others (Young, Klosko, & Weishaar, 2003). Young and colleagues have identified several "early maladaptive schemas" that often underlie cognitions, emotions, and behaviors. For some, the thought change worksheet will have a limited effect until these deeply ingrained patterns of dysfunctional thinking and behavior are addressed. Schemas typically associated with bipolar disorder include defectiveness, failure, unrelenting standards, subjugation, emotional inhibition, and self-sacrifice (Ball et al., 2003). The thoughts and behaviors typically encountered with each of these schemas are as follows (Young, Klosko, & Weishaar, 2003).

DEFECTIVENESS

- Thought—"There is something wrong with me; I am flawed"; "If people get to know me they will not like me."
- Behavior—Insecure around others; hypersensitive to criticism and rejection; avoids sharing concerns or mistakes with others.

FAILURE

- Thought—"I don't measure up; I am stupid, ugly, and less successful than everyone else"; "I have nothing."
- Behavior—Works below ability level; compares own achievement unfavorably to others; might avoid new or difficult tasks; has difficulty setting goals.

UNRELENTING STANDARDS

- Thought—"I can't make any mistakes"; "I will be criticized if I'm not perfect."
- Behavior—Has difficulty relaxing, experiencing a sense of accomplishment, and maintaining satisfying relationships.

SUBJUGATION

- Thought—"I have to put others' needs before mine"; "If I don't give in to others, I might get hurt or abandoned"; "My opinion doesn't really matter."
- Behavior—Easily surrenders control to others and is excessively compliant; chooses controlling partners or avoids relationships altogether.

EMOTIONAL INHIBITION

- Thought—"I must control my emotions so I do not upset anyone'; 'I will lose control if I become emotional."
- Behavior—Inhibits both negative and positive emotions; has difficulty freely expressing genuine feelings; acts in excessively rational and controlled manner.

SELF-SACRIFICE

- Thought—"It doesn't matter if it hurts me, I must do this for him"; "It's more important for me to help others than to worry about my own needs."
- Behavior—Seldom takes care of own needs or seeks out opportunities for self-care and pleasure; always volunteers to help others; may eventually become angry and resentful.

A significant degree of theoretical understanding and supervised training is recommended before attempting to conduct schema therapy in its most comprehensive form. Here it is suggested that the clinician consider the possibility that attitudes related to treatment adherence and impaired psychosocial functioning are associated with early maladaptive beliefs, and help the client become aware of these schemas. Schemas can be specifically targeted using the thought change worksheet by exploring the underlying substance behind the identified "automatic thoughts" in the third column. The goals are to reduce the power of the maladaptive schemas and to promote the development of adaptive schemas through education and challenging dysfunctional beliefs and attitudes. Ball and colleagues (2003) warn that this approach is contraindicated for bipolar clients who are significantly depressed, hypomanic, or manic at the time of treatment, and those who have borderline personality traits or dissociative disorders. Therefore this technique should be used only after the client has achieved a significant degree of stability.

.   .   .

As with many depressed individuals, Mary felt she had little hope for a better future because no matter what she does she can never catch a break. Mary's tendency to live passively and leave things to chance was targeted by helping

TABLE 7.1   Thought Change Worksheet—Major Depression and Bipolar Disorder (Ma)

SITUATION	RESPONSE	AUTOMATIC THOUGHTS
Describe what is (was) going on at the time you experience(d) distress. Who? What? When? Where?	a. What do (did) you feel? b. Use specific emotion words like angry, sad, helpless, scared, hurt, hopeless, disappointed.	a. What was going through mind just before you started feel this way? Any Images? b. Circle the trouble though (the one most connected to the distress).
I was at my apartment today, just lying in my bed, and I was bored. I started to feel like my life was worthless, and I just felt tired of dealing with being bipolar.	Frustrated Angry Hopeless Tired Weak	I will never be well again. *The only way to stop feeling so bad is to end my life.* Nothing I ever do is good enough; I'm a failure. My life is nothing like I want it to be.

her to recognize when her actions influence how she feels. The ACT team workers encouraged Mary to be proactive with her recovery and had her use empowering self-statements to combat her self-defeating thoughts.

The ACT staff also used motivational interviewing strategies with Mary on a regular basis to help her stay engaged in treatment and avoid relapse. By focusing on her values and goals, Mary was able to find the energy and motivation she needed to go to appointments, keep taking her medication, and avoid using alcohol. Also, whenever she began to stay in bed, deviate from her daily schedule, or skip work, the staff used these strategies to help her get back on track by exploring emotional and physical hurdles that were getting in her way.

Mary has been experiencing episodes of depression since she was a teenager, and much of her difficulty is the result of maladaptive schemas, or thought patterns, that developed in the context of a chaotic and sometimes abusive family life. Mary's parents were very critical of her because she did not do well in

ENCE THAT SUPPORTS TROUBLE THOUGHT	EVIDENCE THAT DOES NOT SUPPORT THE TROUBLE THOUGHT	ALTERNATIVE / BALANCED THOUGHTS
e facts that suggest the e thought is true.	List the facts that suggest the trouble thought is not true.	a. Write an alternative or balanced thought considering the facts. b. Rate how much you believe in the alternative or balanced thought (0–10).
e ending life will end in.	There have been several times that I have been symptom free for a little while. I began to feel better when I stopped drinking and was going to meetings. I have been able to work for a while now and usually enjoy it. I had a good time Thursday at the park with Jenny and didn't feel depressed.	Even though I am very depressed and feel miserable right now, there are things I can do to get better, and suicide is not my only option. (8)

school and could not meet the demands they put on her. She began to develop a failure schema that involved thoughts that she could not be good at anything no matter how hard she tried. She also began to believe that her opinion was not as important as others' opinions, and she became excessively compliant and surrendered control to others. The ACT clinician worked with Mary on challenging these thoughts and creating a more balanced and healthier perspective through completing several thought change worksheets (e.g., table 7.1). As she practiced identifying the thoughts that triggered her negative emotions and began to understand their origin, she became more capable of regulating her emotions. This new ability to challenge problematic thinking greatly reduced the intensity and frequency of Mary's depressive symptoms.

8

PTSD and Panic Disorder

James is a 31-year-old single man who has experienced symptoms of PTSD for five years. During his second tour of combat in Afghanistan, he witnessed several of his comrades lose their life when his team was ambushed. James felt helpless as he watched his fellow servicemen strain for their final breaths and simultaneously tried to return shots at the enemy. He managed to find cover during the chaos and was eventually saved by the backup that was called in. James continued to serve his country for three more months before returning home, all the while ceaselessly reviewing the horrific images of that day in his mind. He always felt like the next surprise attack was just around the corner. He did not adjust well to civilian life. He began drinking heavily, and he occasionally used marijuana when he felt the energy to seek out a seller. Nightmares and flashbacks kept James from getting the rest he needed, and this resulted in constant irritability. None of his family or friends could stand to be around him for more than an hour or so. Eventually James's mother persuaded him to see a psychiatrist at the Veterans Administration and he was prescribed Paxil and Restoril. These medications, along with participation in a PTSD group at the VA, have helped James stay relatively stable over the past several years; only once has he required short-term inpatient care. However, three days ago James began to experience an exacerbation of symptoms. He has not been able to leave his home because he feels impending danger all around him. Images of his comrades constantly stream through his mind, and he is emotionally labile. He believes a war movie he recently watched at night may have triggered this acute episode.

PERFORM ASSESSMENT

- Interview
- Suicide/self-harm assessment
- Drug screen
- Crisis action plan
- Safety contract

RELAPSE PREVENTION

- Increase internal LOC
- Motivational enhancement
- Change dysfunctional thinking

RECOVERY PHILOSOPHY

- Client-led treatment
- Utilize/improve personal strengths and resources
- Empowerment
- Prevention and recovery

ESTABLISH EQUILIBRIUM

- Medication adherence
- Feeling safe
- Activity scheduling
- Paradoxical intention
- Exposure
- Dealing with flashbacks/ nightmares

ADDRESS SOCIAL/ ENVIRONMENTAL ISSUES

- Build social supports
- Link to resources
- Change system

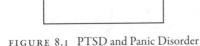

FIGURE 8.1   PTSD and Panic Disorder

*   *   *

Jane is a 42-year-old single woman who lives with her child in a small mobile home in a rural town. She has difficulty leaving the home. Jane is significantly obese and hates being seen by others. Since she was a child, she has been very fearful and cautious, with the expectation that horrible things might happen to her if she is not in a secure place, like her home. In her early twenties she was sexually assaulted by a stranger, and this reinforced her tendency to anticipate negative events. Her anxiety symptoms and accompanying suicidal thoughts have been so debilitating that she has required a total of seventeen months of inpatient treatment beginning at age 25. Occasionally she will muster up enough courage to go to the store or a medical appointment, but she typically avoids crowded places or social activities as much as she can. She describes frequent episodes of panic that include heart palpitations, sweating, shortness of breath, nausea, and chest pain. She relies on others to go places for her and to bring her the things she needs. This dependence on others robs her of the opportunity to challenge her fears and causes significant relationship difficulties as she can often be demanding. Over the past few years she has been self-medicating with a combination of alcohol, benzodiazepines, and sleep aids, such as Benadryl. Recently she has begun refusing to attend her important medical appointments, and her misuse of sedating medications has increased. She claims she is constantly nervous and unable to sleep. She is not considered an imminent danger to herself, and her sister and boyfriend are helping her take care of her child and her home so she does not meet criteria for hospitalization; however, her anxiety issues must be addressed quickly to prevent further decompensation, especially because she has a history of suicidal behavior.

•   •   •

Posttraumatic stress disorder and panic disorder are both anxiety disorders. This chapter focuses on both. Each section first highlights relevant information for PTSD and then shifts to panic disorder.

PTSD can develop in response to several different kinds of trauma. For instance, being in a severe automobile accident, participating in military combat, witnessing a homicide or suicide, experiencing sexual or physical assault, and relentless societal oppression are included among the long list of precipitants. The traumatic event, or series of events, required the individual with PTSD to compensate for a lack of sufficient coping resources in ways that eventually altered various aspects of their biological, psychological, and interpersonal functioning. These changes often manifest through symptoms such as sleep problems or nightmares, hypervigilance, panic attacks, substance abuse, isolation, depression, flashbacks, anger and irritability, dissociation or numbing, and avoidance behavior. An acute episode of symptoms often occurs when the individual is confronted with images, events, or people that trigger emotions that are similar to those felt while experiencing the trauma. Also, increased vulnerability due to substance use or a particularly stressful event or series of events might cause a person with PTSD to decompensate.

Individuals with panic disorder, with or without agoraphobia, can be difficult to treat because many have developed potentially harmful methods of self-medication and there is a high incidence of suicidal behavior.

Many times these individuals are extremely frustrated with their symptoms and are desperate for relief. Unfortunately they may have tried several strategies with limited success, and this can make it difficult for the interventionist to instill hopefulness or optimism. It is important to find out what the person has used in the past to get through episodes of severe anxiety and to determine if he or she was performing these strategies accurately. It could be very upsetting if right away a clinician suggests an intervention that has never worked for the person.

PERFORM ASSESSMENT

Interview*

Clinicians will want to find out what is going on in the client's life currently (major stressors, depression, psychosis, general anxiety, specific phobias, or other things). Also, ask about the duration of their current distress and try to identify a triggering event or set of events that might have caused the increase in symptom severity. Try to identify friends, family members, or mental health service providers they think could help them get through the crisis.

Individuals with schizophrenia, bipolar, major depression, and other diagnoses often have a history of trauma. When a client has a diagnosis of PTSD, it can be difficult to determine which condition is causing the current distress, or to what degree each is contributing. In other words, many times clients who appear depressed are actually struggling with issues of trauma, and clients who present as anxious could be dealing with flashbacks and nightmares from past traumatic experiences rather than their current daily stressors. For these reasons and others, it is important to attempt to find out if the individual has a history of trauma and, if so, whether issues related to the trauma are contributing to the current difficulties.

After it has been established that the client has PTSD or at least a history of significant trauma and is currently dealing with trauma-related issues, clinicians will need to assess the ways in which this is affecting the client. For instance, ask the person what kind of emotions he or she is feeling (sadness, anger, guilt, shame). Also, ask about nightmares and flashbacks (how frequent, how disturbing). Because individuals who have experienced significant trauma often dissociate to cope, find out if the client loses time or has memory problems. Also, ask about feeling numb at times, or if the person tries to feel numb to avoid emotional pain. Ask what events (e.g., anniversary, being alone with a male, driving), people, thoughts, or images trigger a severe emotional response, such as panic. Finally, ask about the ability to sleep (sleeping habits, use of sleep aids). These questions will help to determine which treatment strategies are most appropriate.

The panic disorder assessment should include questions about agoraphobic avoidance, interoceptive avoidance, distraction, and safety behaviors (White & Barlow, 2002). Regarding agoraphobic avoidance, ask the person what he or she is avoiding or too scared to do (e.g., drive a car, go to the store, leave the home, eat). For interoceptive avoidance, ask what physical sensations (e.g., shortness of breath, chest pain, sweating) the individual is experiencing. The fear of these sensations may be causing the avoidance behavior. Next, find out which methods of distraction the individual uses to avoid feeling anxious (e.g., music, TV, talking to someone). These strategies might be helpful for getting through the most acute periods of anxiety, but to prevent it from worsening or occurring repeatedly, the individual must learn to experience the anxiety and overcome it. In other words, the individual should learn to recognize that he or she is not actually in danger, rather than try to feel safe in response to a false threat. To find what safety behaviors the individual is engaging in, ask what he or she does when feeling that a panic or anxiety attack is occurring or is about to occur. For instance, does the person carry a cell phone, require that a certain person be with them, use a food or drink item, or keep medication easily accessible? During a crisis it would not be helpful to eliminate these behaviors; rather, special care should be given to gradually replacing the safety behaviors with more appropriate coping skills (White & Barlow, 2002).

Suicide/Self-harm Assessment*

PTSD and panic disorder can result in severe distress, and suicidal and self-harm behavior is common among those who experience these conditions. Follow the guidelines described in chapter 5 to ensure that an adequate assessment and appropriate intervention is performed. Individuals who have experienced significant trauma, such as sexual abuse, may have a history of cutting or other self-harm behavior. The goal of self-injury is often something other than death. It is important to learn what the behavior does for the client, or at least what he or she is attempting to do, and provide healthy alternative coping strategies. If death is the goal, the process of hospitalization should be initiated.

Drug Screen*

Alcohol abuse is common among those with anxiety disorders. The abuse of prescription medication, such as benzodiazapenes and narcotics, is also prevalent. Unfortunately the combination of these drugs and alcohol can result in death. Therefore even if the client denies substance abuse, education should be provided around the potential consequences of mixing these frequently prescribed medications with alcohol. Review the guidelines for substance use screening provided in chapter 5.

Crisis Action Plan*

Although the crisis action plan should continue to include a specific plan for a psychiatric emergency (i.e., suicidal thoughts, psychotic disturbance, and intense hopelessness), the client with an anxiety disorder will especially benefit from identifying specific triggers and formulating a specific plan for coping with these triggers. As always, the client should be provided with crisis hotline numbers.

Contracts*

The initial contract might target self-harm behavior and abstinence from using substances. Later, contracts might be used to discourage avoidance behavior on the part of the client and enabling behavior by the family or other individuals in the client's life. See the recommendations in the fundamental tools and techniques chapter for engaging the client in this activity.

PTSD

The crisis stabilization worker met with James at his home. James sat with his mother, who was clearly concerned about James's present condition. When James was asked to describe how he had been feeling over the past couple of days, he began to tell about his combat experience and eventually got around to the fact that he felt he was "losing control." He reported not being able to sleep over the past two days because of the "disturbing images" in his head and "intense anxiety that won't seem to go away." The crisis worker asked how long this had been occurring and what he thought might be going on. James said that he had been feeling pretty well until about a week ago, when he started to worry more and felt "more paranoid." He said that things seemed to get really bad after he watched a graphic war movie; this is when the flashbacks became more frequent and obtrusive. The crisis worker asked if he had been seeing a psychologist or psychiatrist and if he was taking medication. James admitted that he missed his last appointment with his psychiatrist and had not been taking his medication over the past three to four weeks. With prompting from his mother, James also admitted that his alcohol consumption had increased over the past month. James was asked if he had recently used any other drugs, to which he responded "no." When the crisis worker asked if he had experienced any thoughts of either hurting himself or ending his life, James became silent then eventually stated that the thought of taking his gun and shooting himself had entered his mind the previous day. However, he quickly explained that he does not want to die and would never kill himself. He denied engaging in any self-harm behavior. The crisis counselor completed the crisis action plan with the help of James and his mother. The counselor pointed out that James needed to contact his psychiatrist to discuss getting back on his medication. James's mother contacted the doctor and scheduled an appointment for the following day. Before the crisis worker left James's home, he prepared a contract that required James to commit to contacting crisis staff if he feels suicidal, to ceasing the use of alcohol, and to allowing his mother to take the ammunition to his gun to her home until he has stabilized. James signed the contract and was provided phone numbers to use in case of an emergency. A follow-up appointment was scheduled for later that day.

PANIC DISORDER

Jane was clearly distressed during the interview, which took place in her home. She was shaking and appeared uncomfortable. At times she became tearful as the interviewer asked her questions about her symptoms and the things going on in her life. Jane explained that over the past couple of weeks she had felt frozen and had not been able to get out of the house. The interviewer asked if she had experienced any recent changes with her family, health, medication, *environment, or other things. Jane reported she had been taking her prescribed medications and several others to sleep. Also, her fear of having a panic attack in public was more intense than it had been in a while. Jane admitted that she was also using alcohol a few times a week, and she showed the staff person the pills she had been taking, so a drug screen was not used.*

Jane reported that she had been feeling depressed because she thinks she is a bad mother and sometimes feels her son would be better off without her. She was asked if she currently had a specific plan to take her own life or hurt herself, and she stated that she did not. To complete the assessment, the interviewer assisted Jane in filling out the crisis action plan. She was able to identify ways in which staff will know when she is doing better or worse, and she expressed her treatment preferences. She also stated that she has tried deep-breathing techniques, but this has not worked for her in the past. When she was asked to describe how she did this, it became clear that her method was incorrect and she agreed to try it again. The treatment phase began once a clear understanding of Jane's clinical difficulties and treatment preferences was established.

ESTABLISH EQUILIBRIUM

Medication Adherence*

It is important to gather information about the individual's current medication use. In some cases increased anxiety and panic attacks may be the result of a recent medication change. At other times it may be the result of an individual's decision to cease taking medications, such as SSRIs, without proper titration. It is also possible that an individual is not taking an anxiety-reducing medication properly.

Affirmations*

Affirmations are positive statements (I am . . . , My . . .) or images (suggesting success, power, health, happiness) that help the client challenge negative, fatalistic thoughts or images and build confidence in their ability to tolerate their various symptoms. The first step is to help the client come up with a phrase or image that is powerful, stands in opposition to a common negative belief or image he or she has, and is something he or she can buy into. Next, encourage the individual to get into the habit of using this affirmation by frequently repeating it throughout the day, especially when feeling poorly. As the client replaces sufferer talk with survivor talk, he or she will begin to feel increasingly more emotionally stable.

Feeling Safe**

PROVIDE EDUCATION*

It is often necessary to educate the client in order to challenge faulty beliefs or help find ways to be safe and feel safe. This might involve researching a particular topic on the Internet to provide more accurate data to the individual. Clinicians may ask clients what people or things help them feel safe and then help them find ways to extend the use of these safety objects or come up with new ones. Some clients need to be taught how to properly identify safety cues in the environment so that they are more confident and competent as they navigate their surroundings (e.g., inform them of places that are typically safe and those that should be avoided as well as red flags that suggest someone does not have their best interest in mind).

DEEP-BREATHING AND RELAXATION STRATEGIES*

This includes monitoring breathing, breathing correctly, imagery, and muscle relaxation (Tsao & Craske, 2000). Typically people who are anxious or tense engage in shallow breathing (short breaths from the chest), which prevents the body from relaxing; they will need to practice breathing in such a way that the abdomen rises instead of the chest. For deep breathing, have the individual get in a relaxed position, place one hand on the abdomen, and take long, deep breathes through the nose and out the mouth. This should continue for as long as it takes to feel relaxed. This activity should be discontinued if the client begins to have difficulty breathing, and extra caution should be used with those with a history of asthma. Clients with PTSD will likely benefit from learning to imagine a safe place while performing relaxation strategies. If the deep-breathing exercise is successful, the clinician can introduce progressive muscle relaxation.

PROGRESSIVE MUSCLE RELAXATION*

Once the individual becomes relaxed and is breathing properly, an instruction is given to tense each muscle group from the feet to the forehead. By purposefully flexing the muscle and then releasing it, one can cause the muscle to become less rigid or strained. As the body relaxes, one's emotional state should become calmer. Additionally, this task requires a certain level of concentration and thus doubles as a distraction technique. Encourage the person to do this regularly for practice and when anxiety is intense to combat tension.

DISTRACTION TECHNIQUES*

Distraction techniques are used for getting through difficult activities when needed (e.g., reading a book or magazine, listening to music, chewing gum or candy, counting). Clients might need help adapting various relaxation and coping strategies to their specific crisis situations.

ASSERTIVENESS TRAINING*

Clients who have experienced trauma might need to learn ways to establish and maintain healthy emotional boundaries so they can have effective relationships and avoid recurring trauma. Reminding clients of their rights and role-playing assertive responses in difficult situations could be an important part of the crisis intervention. This technique could be used early in treatment to help clients disengage from a current stressor as well as later in treatment to build their confidence and competency in avoiding situations that could lead to relapse of a crisis state.

STAYING GROUNDED / MINDFULNESS**

Dissociation can be a troubling symptom of posttraumatic stress. The negative consequences may include forgetting important tasks, relationship problems, confusion, and various other things that cause functional impairment. Therefore it is important that those with PTSD find ways to stay present in the moment, even during times of distress, such as when a negative memory is triggered. The following methods for staying grounded are among those suggested by Williams and Poijula (2002):

- Use all your senses to be aware of your environment.
- Make a plan for the day and let others know what it is.
- Do routine activities in a different way.
- Ask others to help you stay in the present and connected.
- Talk to yourself about what you are experiencing in the present.

Mindfulness is another term used to describe being in the present. According to Linehan (1993b), mindfulness entails successful integration or balance of one's emotional (feeling) and reasonable (intellect) mental states. If a person is predominantly operating in either one of these states, his or her level of functioning is not optimal. When these states are balanced, one is considered to be in a "wise mind" state. When in wise mind, one is better able to handle life's stressors because of an increased awareness of one's emotional state and the ability to accurately assess the situation. Below are some of the skills that Linehan suggests will help clients experience wise mind:

- Experiencing what is happening with awareness; not focusing on how to stop the emotional experience or prolong it. (Encourage the client to try to step away from the event in his or her mind and observe what is going on— dissociation involves stepping away and being unaware of what is going on.)
- Describing events, emotions, and thoughts in words. (This helps the client to determine if what he or she is feeling is what is actually happening. Is there really a threat? What are the facts?)
- Evaluating events, behaviors, and feelings without judging them. (Rather than worrying about whether it is good or bad, just be aware of it.)
- Focusing on events in the present without being distracted by images, thoughts, and feelings involving the past or future.

Activity Scheduling*

To help decrease avoidance behavior, have clients create a list of enjoyable activities they have been avoiding, and help them to reengage in them gradually (create a hierarchical list starting with the easiest and increasing in difficulty). This is a little different from the exposure task because in exposure the clinician might be helping the individual experience something repeatedly until anxiety is reduced. With activity scheduling the goal is to get the individual involved in normal (or desired) daily activities.

Paradoxical Intention**

Paradoxical intention is a brief therapeutic strategy developed by Victor Frankl (2006) for treating obsessive-compulsive and phobic conditions, especially those with underlying anticipatory anxiety. The individual is asked to intentionally attend to, even if for a short time, the thing he or she fears. According to Frankl, "This procedure consists of a reversal of the patient's attitude, inasmuch as his fear is replaced by a paradoxical wish. By this treatment, the wind is taken out of the sails of the anxiety" (124). In practical terms clinicians will ask the individual who begins to have panic symptoms in response to a feared event to try to have the panic response without the event. By purposefully attempting to feel that which one fears feeling, there is an attitude change, and now the client is working on decreasing anticipatory anxiety. This method works best with certain personality types, especially those who are willing to find a little humor in their behavior. If the person is not likely to engage in this activity lightheartedly, the likelihood of success is low.

Exposure Therapy***

The goal of exposure therapy (ET) is for the individual to habitually be exposed to and overcome a fear-producing stimulus. This includes exposing the person to the physical arousal alone and to the physical arousal during an actual feared activity. Through this process the individual builds self-confidence and a sense of mastery over the stimulus (Pollard & Zuercher-White, 2003). Livanou (2001:181) explains the alternative to direct exposure: "In the treatment of PTSD, imaginal exposure involves the trauma survivor or the therapist narrating repeatedly the traumatic experience in detail and in the present tense, while the survivor is focusing on the most distressing aspects of the trauma until habituation occurs. Distress and its reduction during imaginal exposure is monitored."

The safest method is a gradual approach that includes breaking down very difficult tasks into smaller, more manageable tasks. Spend as much time as possible (through repetition or sustained duration) exposing the individual to the stimulus while encouraging relaxation. Avoidance behavior must eventually be completely stopped for a full recovery, but this may not be achievable in the time spent with the individual. In fact, this is not really the focus in crisis intervention. The main goal of this strategy is to help the individual return to his or her precrisis level of functioning as stress relief and the ability to engage in activities of daily living begin.

Dealing with Flashbacks and Nightmares***

To address problematic flashbacks and nightmares associated with PTSD, it may be helpful to use a strategy called "rewriting the script." Just as one might reframe a statement to make it more pleasant, it is possible to manipulate the content of a flashback or nightmare to make it less emotionally disturbing. We all have the power to choose whether or not to believe something (e.g., others' opinions, our health status, our safety) as well as the power to convince ourselves to believe something other than our immediate perception. Some people, especially those who are more flexible and imaginative, can take a negative thought or image and transform it into a more positive or healthy one through various mental processes. To rewrite the script, have the client write down (or verbally describe) the flashback or nightmare, then provide assistance to the client in creating an ending to the event that produces feelings of safety, empowerment, or optimism. The client will need to come up with an ending that is acceptable and believable (i.e., is reality based and relevant) for it to have an impact. This process will need to be repeated for the same flashback or nightmare, and for new ones, until they can be effectively managed. If practiced frequently and correctly, this exercise should improve reality-testing and problem-solving skills besides reducing negative emotions associated troubling images and dreams.

PTSD

The crisis counselor met with James later in the evening and checked on his compliance with the safety contract. He had given his gun to his mom and refrained from using alcohol. He also denied having thoughts of harming himself. The counselor spent a few minutes educating James about PTSD, focusing on the fact that his strong emotions are likely associated with images related to his combat experience, and explained that over the next few days the crisis staff would be helping him learn ways to cope with the anxiety he experiences as well as challenge the thought process that causes him to feel paranoid. The counselor discussed the various coping skills with James and had him add the ones he felt most comfortable with to his crisis action plan. These were self-soothing with music, meditation, and taking a hot shower to relax. James was also guided through the deep-breathing and progressive muscle relaxation sequence to ensure he could do this correctly. Although he thought these activities were awkward, he was encouraged to practice each several times a day, especially at night before attempting to sleep.

Over the next two days James was encouraged to practice relaxation strategies with positive affirmations with the theme that he is safe. He was encouraged to continue to think of the coping strategies that have helped in the past as well as the ways in which he can begin to try the new ones he had just learned. The crisis counselor also took James to some of the places that he enjoys visiting (the park, the beach) to improve his mood and help decrease isolation and avoidance. Because James has not been sleeping, the crisis counselor helped him develop a daily schedule to promote better sleep. This included exercising for at least one hour inside or outside the home, avoiding afternoon naps, stopping consumption of caffeinated beverages in the evening, and going to bed at 9:00 each night. James was provided education about his medication and was monitored for adherence each day.

A daily journal was a key factor in James's stability. Although some clients are not interested in or capable of writing in a journal, James was, and this was fully utilized. He was encouraged to practice mindfulness by writing detailed accounts of his activities, thoughts, and feelings each day. He was also asked to write a positive affirmation at the end of each journal entry. He usually wrote something like, "I am safe, I have nothing to fear right now." James's flashbacks and nightmares were also targeted with the journal. He was asked to describe the experience in his journal and to complete the entry with a healthy alternate ending and positive affirmation.

.   .   .

To provide quick relief of her symptoms and to help her regain control over her emotions, Jane was taught coping skills. She was told that the more she fights against having anxiety, the more intense it becomes, and she was encouraged to try to accept that anxiety is all right. She was instructed to imagine she is floating on top of the wave of anxiety instead of pushing against it. Jane was also taught the other ways to cope with distress, and special emphasis was placed on maintaining proper sleep hygiene so that Jane would become less dependent on sleep aids. She was encouraged to begin taking only her prescribed medication to prevent overdose and to help her psychiatrist make an accurate assessment of her medication needs.

Jane was also provided with psychoeducation about panic disorder. The clinician explained to her how panic results from a brief burst of adrenaline in the body. This adrenaline results in shortened breaths and rapid heart beating that is often mistaken for a heart attack. Once Jane understood the physiology behind panic attacks, she was able to acknowledge that it was a biological reaction and did not mean she was dying. She also understood that taking deep diaphragmatic breaths helped her relax and counter the panic symptoms, because it is impossible for her to be both anxious and relaxed at the same time.

Jane had been avoiding leaving her home, and this had to be addressed soon because the more she avoids, the more anxiety she will feel, and she will continue to experience increased difficulty with getting out of her home as this cycle continues. Staff created an activity schedule with Jane that gradually built up to her going to appointments. This process was broken down into ten steps, beginning with imagining going outside and using relaxation strategies to calm her anxiety. Jane practiced pairing a variety of distraction and relaxation strategies with her thoughts of going outside until she found one that was helpful. She voiced several concerns about what people will say and do to her if they see her, and many of these things were unrealistic. Education was provided to challenge these thoughts. Also, Jane's assertiveness was targeted by teaching her various social skills, such as effective communication, and she was informed that she has rights as a human being; if people do not respect these rights they are wrong, and she can let them know. Jane slowly built confidence in her ability to tolerate social activities, and her anxious and depressive symptoms began to decrease to a point where she felt emotionally and physically stable.

ADDRESS SOCIAL AND ENVIRONMENTAL ISSUES

General Tips*

When working with clients who have anxiety disorders, clinicians should be careful to not be excessively protective by eliminating all stressors in the client's environment. Sometimes the line between helping and enabling is difficult to recognize when working with severely anxious individuals. The key is to identify issues that will likely cause chronic stress despite clients' efforts to improve their coping ability, and to help problem solve them. These chronically stressful issues might include abusive relationships, a dangerous or unhealthy housing situation, and lack of financial resources. Clinicians will likely need to involve community supports, such as social services, the police department, or a domestic violence shelter, in resolving these issues. An example of enabling would be soliciting friends, family, or neighbors to run errands for the client so that he or she does not have to experience the stress of leaving home or being in public. Additionally, follow the general recommendations in chapter 5 for addressing social and environmental stressors.

Change the System**

It may be necessary to include the family or social network in the intervention process. The individual in crisis will likely benefit from having those around them be more knowledgeable and sympathetic to the individual's difficulty. Furthermore, they can act as cotherapists by reinforcing the strategies the individual has been learning. For example, family members can encourage the individual to engage in activities and decrease avoidance behavior rather than do things for him or her. Often family members try to be supportive by giving in to the wishes of the individual. This might involve making excuses for missed appointments, going to the store for the person, or driving the person places (Wolfe, 2005). Family members need to know that this can exacerbate the problem, and the intervention staff can empower them to change their response to the individual. They will likely be relieved to know that they do not necessarily need to alter their lifestyle to wait on the client hand and foot. Many times this transition can be difficult for family members who have become codependent; thus clinicians should confront them carefully and empathically.

PTSD

James does not have an adequate support system because his family and friends have distanced themselves from him over the past year. Also, James has lost much of his confidence in being able to perform in social situations as his interpersonal skills have become rusty because he has lived as a shut-in. To address these issues, the crisis counselor began to take advantage of opportunities to teach and model assertiveness, communication, and other social skills. James was escorted to various socially active places like the grocery store and mall to practice his skills and become better able to tolerate situations with a high level of stimuli.

To improve his support system, James's mother was asked to meet the counselor at James's home to discuss the reasons why family and friends began to avoid contact with him. It became evident that James frequently became excessively emotional when there was a disagreement or when he felt that others were accusatory. The counselor explained that the intense emotions could be related to high levels of stress, and this could partially be resolved with continued use of coping skills and other strategies. The counselor helped James role-play various interactions with his family and friends and helped him practice effective communication and emotion regulation. James was also introduced to a local support group for anxiety sufferers so that he can receive more support and have another outlet for socialization.

•   •   •

Jane had a boyfriend who stayed with her much of the time. He was a kindhearted person who became distressed when Jane seemed upset. To make sure she stayed comfortable and did not become upset, he tirelessly addressed her every need to the best of his ability. He drove places for her, talked to people for her, and scrambled to get her whatever she requested to keep her calm. When he had to work, her mother took over this role. Jane's system of family and friends was enabling her to engage in an extreme level of avoidance behavior, which had to stop if she was ever going to recover from panic attacks and agoraphobia. With Jane's permission the program staff met with her and her boyfriend and mother on two occasions to educate them about Jane's condition and to ask them to encourage Jane to practice using the deep-breathing and other skills. They were also shown a copy of Jane's activity schedule, and they agreed to encourage her to do more as they did less.

RELAPSE PREVENTION

To prepare clients for future success in managing their symptoms, underlying issues such as lack of motivation, feelings of helplessness and hopelessness, cognitive distortion, and maladaptive behaviors may need to be addressed. Individuals experiencing panic disorder will likely be committing "probability errors" and "severity errors" that need to be corrected. Probability errors involve an overestimation of the likelihood of having a panic or symptom attack. Severity errors involve catastrophic thinking or the belief that the symptoms of the attack will be unbearable. The goal is to reduce the occurrence of these errors and to increase feelings of self-confidence in coping with feared situations. Clinicians can help the individual maintain a feeling of control by helping them learn to challenge negative automatic thoughts. The following interventions address these factors. These strategies are typically used once the individual is stable with the goal of maintaining treatment gains and increasing recovery skills, but they may need to be used early in the intervention if the client is having difficulty committing to making necessary changes.

Increase Internal Locus of Control*

Many people who experience chronic anxiety have an external locus of control. They feel their ability to influence situations in their life is limited, and therefore they feel vulnerable. This often leads to constant worry as well as dependence on others. This intervention could be used throughout the course of treatment. With every effort the client makes to overcome fears during the treatment process, point out the relationship between actions and the relative impact in the world.

Motivation Enhancement*

Clients who experience panic disorder, agoraphobia, PTSD, and other anxiety disorders often struggle with the difficult treatment process. With many strategies, clients are asked to face their fears before they can actually experience relief. It will be beneficial to become familiar with the motivation enhancement techniques to prepare clients for treatment and to maintain their motivation throughout.

Change Dysfunctional Thinking**

One of the primary treatment goals is to help the individual become more rational. This is done by challenging unrealistic thoughts about present danger or capacity to handle various situations. The thought change worksheet is a great tool for increasing rational and positive thinking. The more clients practice this activity daily, the sooner they will regain control over their emotions.

The first step is to identify the situation or stimuli to which the individual is responding. Sometimes anxiety attacks or dissociative symptoms may seem to occur randomly, and the individual might have difficulty providing a specific situation or trigger. Other times the individual can give an exact description of an activity that prompts an anxious reaction. Next, identify the specific emotional reaction to the stressor. Assist the individual in identifying the specific feelings that are provoked so that he or she can better communicate feelings to others and better track the ability to manage symptoms.

An example of the coping statement written at the end of the thought change worksheet might be "I feel very nervous and scared right now, but I know I am not in danger; it is just the way my body has learned to respond to stress, and it will eventually become less sensitive." This stands in sharp contrast to the dysfunctional language that likely dominates during times of crises, such as "This is unbearable and there is nothing I can do."

Another benefit of the thought change worksheet is that it helps the individual focus on the present experience. Many times individuals who experience anxiety will easily shift their attention to "what-if" scenarios when they begin to think of a feared situation (Wolfe, 2005). This speculation about potential negative outcomes only increases anxiety and keeps the individual from resolving triggered arousal effectively.

Other tips. Help the client continue to engage in the activities listed in the activity schedule. Those who are able may want to keep a log or journal of their activities; others may simply want to tell someone close to encourage or challenge them when they begin to engage in avoidance behavior. Also, do not let a recurrence of a panic or symptom attack put the individual back at square one. Help the person realize the time that went by without one and the fact that he or she survived it, and then assist with engaging in regular activities as soon as possible.

PTSD

After James was fairly stable and had begun taking his prescribed medication consistently, the intervention began to focus on relapse prevention. To start, the crisis counselor assisted James in shifting from an external locus of control to an internal one. This involved pointing out the several areas of his life that demonstrate his actions are meaningful and powerful. James was able to state that much of the time he feels powerless and thinks that his efforts at a better life are futile because he is just unlucky. The counselor used the example of James's current participation in treatment and resulting improvement to show that he does have control and can make positive changes.

Since part of the reason James began to decompensate was the inability to stay engaged in treatment, motivational interviewing strategies were used to increase his level of commitment to the recovery process. The counselor helped him address through discussion and problem solving various reasons he was not confident in his ability to recover. James was asked to look forward and see the benefits of staying compliant with treatment and pushing himself to be more active. This seemed to improve his attitude regarding group attendance, taking his medications, and seeing his psychiatrist regularly.

Finally, James was taught how to use a thought change worksheet to challenge stress provoking thoughts (table 8.1). The crisis counselor did five of these with James throughout the treatment process, and they were effective in reducing his negative emotions. It was explained to James that the better he gets at challenging destructive thoughts and reframing them in a balanced way, the more control he will have over his emotions. James was provided several copies of the worksheet and was encouraged to practice using this tool daily.

· · · ·

Jane's expectations about what might happen to her in public were unrealistic. Staff used psychoeducation to help her realize that the probability and potential severity of the things she feared were exaggerated. The thought change worksheet was used to help Jane challenge these errors in thinking (table 8.2). Although she struggled to find evidence that did not support her panic-related thoughts, eventually she was able to point out the flaws in her thinking, and her anxious feelings began to weaken. Jane also held a strong belief that she had little control over the events in her life. This external locus of control contributed to her sense of hopelessness and helplessness. To address this, staff worked with her on recognizing all the ways in which she does in fact exert control in her life. Also, she was encouraged to write empowering self-statements and to display these around her home. As Jane began to make progress, there was some concern that her motivation to refrain from falling back into old habits was waning. Motivational interviewing strategies were employed to

TABLE 8.1 Thought Change Worksheet—PTSD (James)

SITUATION	RESPONSE	AUTOMATIC THOUGHTS	EVIDENCE THAT SUPPORTS THE TROUBLE THOUGHT	EVIDENCE THAT DOES NOT SUPPORT THE TROUBLE THOUGHT	ALTERNATIVE / BALANCED THOUGHTS
Describe what is (was) going on at the time you experience(d) distress. Who? What? When? Where?	a. What do (did) you feel? b. Use specific emotion words like angry, sad, helpless, scared, hurt, hopeless, disappointed.	a. What was going through your mind just before you started to feel this way? Any Images? b. Circle the trouble thought (the one most connected to the distress).	List the facts that suggest the trouble thought is true.	List the facts that suggest the trouble thought is not true.	a. Write an alternative or balanced thought considering the facts. b. Rate how much you believe in the alternative or balanced thought (0–10).
On Saturday morning I was at home by myself and I thought I saw three men outside my window pointing at me. It was like they were getting ready to break through my door and try to kill me or something.	Angry Worried Terrified Confused	I had a flashback of the war when I felt stuck in the hole hiding. I am going to die because I do not have my gun. I wondered if they were just neighbors or if they were here to get me. People are always out to hurt me and I can never feel safe.	It is very difficult for me to feel safe and calm because of my PTSD. I live in a neighborhood that has a pretty high crime rate. When I was in combat many people were trying to kill me. I worry about my safety constantly.	Nothing bad has actually happened to me since I've been home. I am not longer in a war situation. There are times that I have felt safe enough to leave the house and do whatever I want.	There are enough good people out there who would help me if something were to happen. Even though I worry, the truth is that no one has harmed me since I've been home. (7)

TABLE 8.2 Thought Change Worksheet—Panic Disorder (Jane)

SITUATION	RESPONSE	AUTOMATIC THOUGHTS	EVIDENCE THAT SUPPORTS THE TROUBLE THOUGHT	EVIDENCE THAT DOES NOT SUPPORT THE TROUBLE THOUGHT	ALTERNATIVE / BALANCED THOUGHTS
Describe what is (was) going on at the time you experience(d) distress. Who? What? When? Where?	a. What do (did) you feel? b. Use specific emotion words like angry, sad, helpless, scared, hurt, hopeless, disappointed.	a. What was going through your mind just before you started to feel this way? Any Images? b. Circle the trouble thought (the one most connected to the distress).	List the facts that suggest the trouble thought is true.	List the facts that suggest the trouble thought is not true.	a. Write an alternative or balanced thought considering the facts. b. Rate how much you believe in the alternative or balanced thought (0–10).
Me and my case worker at my home as I was getting ready to go to Dr. Morgan's office on Tuesday morning. I began feeling like I was going to be sick. All I could think about was all of the people at the doctor's office staring at me and talking about me.	Fear Panic Frustration Weakness Worry Nervousness	People are going to laugh at me and call me names. I can't do anything on my own. I'm so fat and hideous looking. I'm going to be trapped in that office with all of those mean people and who knows what they will do to me. I just want to stay home.	I usually become anxious around other people. I have to stay for the appointment or Dr. Morgan will stop seeing me. I probably won't know any of the people there.	The secretary let me wait on the porch one time. I met some nice people there one time when I went to a group. Dr. Morgan wouldn't let them hurt me. There are several doors to go out in case I get scared, and Judy (the secretary) likes me.	I have to go to my appointment today even if it is very difficult. If there are a bunch of mean people there who want to make fun of me, I'm sure Judy and Dr. Morgan will help me and I can sit outside the office if I have to. (8)

help her stay focused and interested in recovery. Staff frequently had Jane talk about the benefits of achieving her goals. Also, she was asked to identify any barriers to treatment or anything that was causing her to feel less confident about her ability to overcome severe anxiety. She eventually felt stable enough to leave her home and attend her appointments; she was no longer in an acute stage of her illness, and her overall level of functioning increased after crisis intervention.

9

Substance-Related Disorders

Tina is 26-year-old woman who entered a crisis stabilization and detoxification program because of recent binging with alcohol and cocaine as well as an increase in risky behaviors such as driving while intoxicated, falling asleep while cooking, and mixing various prescription medications. Tina has been diagnosed with polysubstance dependence and major depressive disorder. She also has received a diagnosis of dependent personality disorder. She lives with her boyfriend and does not work; she receives financial support from her parents and her boyfriend. She recently applied for assistance with obtaining employment through a vocational rehabilitation program, but a positive drug screen caused her application to be denied. Tina has never been arrested for a drug-related charge, but she has been in several fights and has been seriously injured a few times. For various reasons Tina's substance use has increased over the past month, and she has become emotionally unstable.

•   •   •

When assessing an individual with substance-related issues it is necessary to ask about mood, psychotic, anxiety, and other symptoms because substance abuse and other mental illnesses often occur together. When clients reports anxiety, it is important to ask about the concerns they have and whether their safety is in jeopardy. When a client is significantly depressed, the assessment should include a discussion about suicidal ideation and behavior. It can be difficult to determine if the client is actually experiencing two different conditions because cocaine and amphetamine use and the withdrawal from other substances can cause symptoms that might mimic

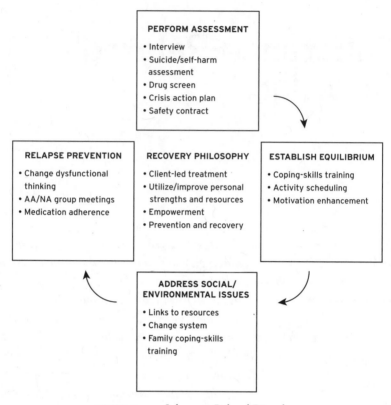

FIGURE 9.1   Substance-Related Disorders

anxiety, psychosis, mania, or depressive symptoms. Either way, these symptoms can be addressed during the intervention. The need for medical treatment, such as detoxification, should also be assessed. This is typically necessary for those who drink heavily every day and users of opiates such as heroin. It is also helpful to assess the client's current level of motivation to stop using substances.

PERFORM ASSESSMENT

Interview*

One of the initial tasks when working with someone who is abusing substances, along with assessing risk for harming self or others, is assessing the motivation to stop. This assessment will help to determine how much time needs to be spent on motivation-enhancing activities versus more coping-focused or problem-solving ones. The idea is that if the person does not want to make changes, he or she will not be responsive to any of the suggestions offered. The stages of change, described by Prochaska and DiClemente (1984) in their transtheoretical model, can be used to identify a client's current level of motivation to reduce drug or alcohol use. These stages of change include precontemplation, contemplation, preparation, action, and maintenance. Motivational interviewing strategies are designed primarily to move those in the first two stages further along the change process.

Clients who enter treatment and are content with the status quo, often called "precontemplators," will fail to make progress regardless of the clinician's skill level. As DiClemente and Velasquez (2002:202–3) have stated, "Precontemplators do not want to be lectured to or given 'action' techniques when they are not ready to change." Those who are more ambivalent about making changes in their behavior are in the contemplation stage. These clients are aware of the arguments to stop using, but they are not sure that the benefits of sobriety outweigh the costs.

DiClemente and Velasquez (2002) offer suggestions on how to tailor interventions to the client's readiness to change. In the first stage, precontemplation, there are those who are reluctant, rebellious, resigned, or rationalizing. Those who are unaware of, or not interested in changing, their behavior (reluctant) may find nonthreatening empathic listening and feedback most helpful. For those who present as hostile and resistant (rebellious), describe the change options (slow and incremental, complete abstinence) and treatment strategies (individual therapy, support groups) that are available and express agreement in the fact that only they can change their behavior. For those who seem to lack the energy or confidence to make changes (resigned) it will be helpful to work on instilling hope and exploring barriers to change. For clients who consider their problematic behavior either the fault of someone else or not as severe as others may think (rationalizing), it is important not to become engaged in argument. Instead, provide empathic listening and acknowledge the positive consequences of drug or alcohol use while also encouraging exploration of the negative consequences.

Individuals in the second stage of change are called "contemplators." These clients may be more receptive to receiving education and exploring their thoughts and feelings about their behavior. Strategies that increase self-efficacy and self-confidence can be helpful for these clients. Also, the clinician should reflect and elicit change-talk (e.g., "If I stopped drinking I would feel less guilty around my family"; "I know I can stop using cocaine again") from the client. The overall goal is to tip the balance in favor of making necessary changes (DiClemente and Velasquez, 2002).

Suicide/Self-harm Assessment*

Even if a substance-related disorder is their primary illness, clients with these conditions often have comorbid anxiety or mood disorders. Thus the suicide assessment is still relevant and important. Furthermore, use of substances is a significant risk factor for completed suicide. Follow the recommendations outlined in chapter 5 to complete the assessment.

Drug Screen*

The drug screen is most salient when treating someone with a known substance-related disorder. The use of instruments such as breathalyzers or urine drug screens can provide a more accurate assessment of current use. Additionally, daily screenings may help the client feel more accountable for his or her actions. It is important to obtain an accurate assessment of the frequency and quantity of substance use so that appropriate referrals for a higher level of care can be made if necessary.

Crisis Action Plan*

When working with individuals who are abusing substances, it might be more helpful to call the crisis action plan a "relapse action plan." The plan should include specific information about various triggers and specific coping strategies to use when confronted with a trigger. As with other conditions, an important issue to address with substance-abusing clients is harm reduction. For instance, individuals who are mixing substances should be discouraged from doing this. If necessary, some prescription medications (e.g., benzodiazepines) should be taken away if the client is likely to continue using alcohol. If a client has a support system, these persons should be utilized as much as possible to help provide encouragement and monitoring. The client should also be provided with crisis hotline numbers and a list of coping strategies.

Contracts*

Contracts can be used to increase accountability and to give the client specific instruction on how to reduce or cease substance use. The contract might include various people or places the client should avoid. It can also provide a list of alternative coping skills that the client agrees to use during times of distress.

* * *

During the initial intake assessment the therapist began by telling Tina about the program she had been referred to and explained the need to obtain accurate information from her. Tina was anxious about being away from her home and was reluctant to cooperate because she did not feel she really needed treatment. She said she was staying at the center only because her boyfriend told her she couldn't come back until she got help. The therapist began to ask Tina about her past substance use and then turned to her recent use. Tina described without reservation several years of alcohol and other drug use beginning when she was 13 years old, but she was more hesitant to discuss her more recent behavior. The therapist explained that honesty would make the process go faster and then used screening questionnaires to help illicit more detailed information. Tina admitted to using alcohol every day for most of the day as well as cocaine, prescription pain medication, and Xanax or Klonopin whenever she was able to obtain it. She was later required to participate in a urine drug screen as part of the center's standard protocol. The therapist asked how she was able to get the drugs since she is not working, and she stated that her parents give her money when she asks for it.

The therapist then focused on Tina's emotional functioning and asked about symptoms of depression and anxiety. Tina stated that for over a month she had been feeling hopeless because of failed efforts to obtain work. Additionally, her boyfriend had given her an ultimatum: she could either help with rent and other expenses or leave. Tina stated that she was feeling terrible and didn't know what else to do, so she began drinking heavily and doing whatever else she could to numb her feelings. The therapist asked Tina if she had also engaged in self-injury; she replied that she used to but had not done that in a while. On further investigation it became clear that a second goal of her increased substance use was to get the attention of her boyfriend and parents and to show them she is not feeling well. Tina denied having thoughts of ending her life and stated that she has never attempted suicide.

The assessment concluded with the completion of the crisis action plan. Tina was asked to describe her behavior and appearance when she is feeling well versus not well, and she was asked about whom she wanted to be involved in her treatment as well as what kinds of treatment she prefers. She stated that she does not like group therapy because she is shy, and she identified various medications that she prefers over others. Tina was asked to think of coping strategies other than drug use that she has found helpful in the past. She listed reading and taking a hot shower on her action plan, and the therapist was able to locate some books for her. The rules of the treatment program were read to her, and she agreed to not use substances while receiving treatment. Tina was then seen by the nurse and psychiatrist and shown to her room.

ESTABLISH EQUILIBRIUM

Several different strategies have been proven effective for helping addicts reduce substance use. The first phase of the intervention includes teaching new coping skills and enhancing the client's motivation to engage in the treatment process and make necessary behavioral changes. These strategies are described below.

Coping and Social Skills Training*

EDUCATION*

- Describe the typical symptoms of substance abuse and dependence (e.g., problems in daily functioning, failed attempts to cease or reduce use, lying to family or friends, tolerance, withdrawal).
- Discuss normal or healthy versus problem drinking.
- Assist the client in identifying precipitants to binge episodes, lapse, relapse, etc.
- Explore the role of inactivity, peers, distress, and mental health issues in substance use.

COPING SKILLS*

Help the client find ways to get through stressful moments by discussing distraction and self-soothing techniques such as meditating, praying, reading, listening to music, going for a walk, exercising, or visiting a friend.

DEEP BREATHING*

This includes monitoring breathing, breathing correctly, and imagery (Tsao & Craske, 2000). For deep breathing, have the individual get in a relaxed position, place one hand on the abdomen, and take long, deep breaths through the nose and out the mouth. Many people do not breathe correctly, so they may need to practice breathing in such a way that the abdomen rises instead of the chest.

PROGRESSIVE MUSCLE RELAXATION*

Once the individual becomes relaxed and is breathing properly, give the instruction to tense then relax each muscle group from the feet to the forehead. By purposefully tensing the muscle then releasing it, one can make the muscle less tense. Encourage the person to do this regularly for practice and when anxiety, anger, or frustration is intense to combat tension.

ASSERTIVENESS TRAINING*

Assertiveness training can be used to help clients develop effective drink- or drug-refusing strategies. They need to know they have the right to be healthy, even if peers or family members prefer that they do not change. It is not enough to just tell a substance abuser to stay away from people who contribute to their use. They often need help with communicating their intentions clearly and in a way that will not sever the relationship. Practice multiple hypothetical scenarios to increase the chances that they will say no when they need to.

PROBLEM-SOLVING TRAINING*

Explain that it is necessary to be flexible, be persistent (don't easily give up on negotiation), separate feelings from the issue, and not get caught in the blame game (McKay, Fanning, & Paleg, 1994). Use role-playing and discussion about real or hypothetical scenarios to help guide the client through problem-solving steps: defining problem, generating possible solutions, assessing pros and cons of each solution, choosing the best solution, and carrying out the plan (Miklowitz, 2002).

ACTIVITY SCHEDULING*

Boredom is one the most common triggers for drug and alcohol use relapse. The first step in increasing activity is to create a pleasurable activities checklist. Have the client think about the things he or she likes to do (e.g., walking, talking with friends and family, going to the park, watching action movies, cooking) and then write them down on a piece of paper. Next, go through the list and discuss specific ways to begin incorporating these activities into a daily schedule. It is important that a realistic plan is developed and that the necessary supports are in place to prevent failed attempts. The second aspect of activity scheduling is to create a daily activity log. This journal of attempted activities will provide accountability as well as a way to monitor which activities are helpful in keeping the client away from high-risk situations.

MOTIVATION ENHANCEMENT**

One of the primary goals of substance abuse treatment is to encourage commitment to making necessary changes. It can be very difficult to combat the urge to use the drug one is addicted to; therefore motivation must remain high. If the clinician is trying much harder than the individual being helped, it is often necessary to change gears and use motivational interviewing strategies. Not only will this make the current intervention easier and more effective, but it will help sustain the person's dedication to make life changes and continue the treatment process after the acute episode is over. Through motivational interviewing (Miller & Rollnick, 2002), the client will explore the ambivalence he or she experiences regarding change, improve the commitment to the change process, and become prepared to take maximum advantage of treatment. Use the instructions provided in chapter 5 to engage the client in a motivational interview.

•   •   •

Tina's treatment began with several sessions that focused on improving her coping and social skills. The therapist taught each of the coping skills (relaxation, problem solving, etc.) and asked the center's support staff to assist with reinforcing daily use through reminders and praise. The therapist spent significant time teaching assertiveness and problem-solving skills and used role-playing of various scenarios to help Tina become competent with these skills. She was also encouraged to develop a repertoire of self-soothing strategies to use when she is upset or feeling low. In one session Tina was provided a sheet of paper with a printed weekly calendar on it and was assisted in completing an activity schedule that she can begin using upon discharge.

Three days into Tina's stay at the crisis center, she was still just going through the motions and did not seem interested in making a serious commitment to change. She became more emotionally stable because of the structured environment, medications, and abstinence from drugs, but she was still difficult to engage in serious discussion about her problematic lifestyle. The therapist used motivation-interviewing strategies during two sessions to boost Tina's commitment to make necessary changes in her life. Although it was difficult for her, Tina was able to identify various goals for her life and to explore ways in which her substance use has prevented her from achieving these goals. Her sense of the importance of stopping drug use as well as her confidence in being able to develop a drug-free lifestyle increased, and the therapist continued to illicit change-talk during the remainder of her stay at the center.

ADDRESS SOCIAL AND ENVIRONMENTAL ISSUES

General Tips*

When working with chronic substance abusers, clinicians will find that many individuals who have been in and out of drug and alcohol treatment programs are familiar with the phrase "people, places, and things." This phrase is used in support groups because in most cases it is the key to recovery. Clients need help using their coping, problem-solving, and assertiveness skills to effectively put this common mantra into daily practice. This can be a difficult part of the intervention for clients who are faced with the need to end long-term relationships, relocate, or withdraw from social norms. Follow the general tips for altering the social environment as described in chapter 5.

Family Coping Skills Training**

In many cases, especially when the client is married or living with parents, it will be necessary to address issues within the family system. This might involve educating family members about the negative consequences of their enabling behavior. This discussion should be followed by teaching assertiveness skills so that family members can begin to break their problematic habits. Also, problem-solving, coping, and communication skills, such as those described in the individual coping skills section, should be taught to family members where indicated. As each member of the family unit becomes more emotionally healthy and knowledgeable about the client's needs, the likelihood of stabilization and sobriety will increase.

•   •   •

During the assessment Tina reported that her parents are financially supporting her and admitted that they give her money anytime she requests it. The therapist told Tina that the center likes to involve the family in the treatment process when it seems appropriate and asked her to give permission to contact them. After the pros and cons of family involvement were discussed, Tina eventually decided to allow the therapist to contact her parents and invite them to attend one or two sessions. Tina's parents came the following evening, and the therapist provided education about Tina's condition and what they can do to help her. Most important, the therapist explained how they are enabling her to use substances. They were encouraged to begin to allow Tina to suffer the natural consequences of her behavior and to limit financial assistance. They also agreed to stop giving Tina cash and instead pay bills directly with her until she is able to obtain employment.

Tina stated one of the primary stressors in her life is her tumultuous relationship with her boyfriend. She has been with him for several years and has no intention of leaving him, but she would like to improve the way they interact. The boyfriend was invited to attend a session and came the following afternoon. The therapist reviewed the communication and problem-solving skills and allowed Tina and her boyfriend to practice them. Another issue that needed to be addressed was Tina's problematic relationship with a close friend who often assisted her with obtaining drugs. The therapist encouraged Tina to establish clear boundaries with this friend and used assertiveness training to prepare her for this.

RELAPSE PREVENTION

Refer to Twelve-Step Programs*

Twelve-step programs, or other support groups, can be the most important recovery tool for some clients. This treatment modality should be suggested for most individuals who struggle with addiction. The key is to help find a group that is convenient for them to attend and one that they feel connected to. There are a number of excuses for not attending that the client might offer (e.g., I don't want to hear about people's problems, I don't have a car, I don't need that); however, the client should still be encouraged to give group attendance a fair trial. The more meetings the client can attend the better, but the level of participation may vary depending on employment and family status, among other things.

Medication Adherence*

When helping individuals who abuse substances, it is important to inform prescribing physician(s) about the substance use so that lethal interactions between street and prescribed drugs do not occur. In many, but not all, cases the client will be permitted to continue taking medications as prescribed while being encouraged to cease alcohol and drug use. Also, if the client is abusing prescribed medication, communication among all treatment providers will help limit the client's ability to manipulate the system and will increase the chances of developing a solid treatment plan. Follow the recommendations for improving medication adherence provided in chapter 5.

Change Dysfunctional Thinking**

The substance-related disorder thought change worksheet in appendix B varies somewhat from the thought change worksheet used with other disorders. It can be used to help the substance-abusing client to identify high-risk situations and generate alternative responses to triggers, which is one of the keys to relapse prevention (Blume & Marlatt, 2009; Marlatt and Gordon, 1985). The first step is to clearly identify the scenarios that illicit thoughts of using alcohol, cocaine, marijuana, and so forth. Ask the client to identify past and recent situations that eventually led to substance use.

TABLE 9.1   Thought Change Worksheet—Substance Abuse (Tina)

TRIGGER SITUATION	RESPONSE	SUBSTANCE USE BEHAVIOR	POSITIVE AND NEGATIVE CONSEQUENCES
Who? What? When? Where?	a. What do (did) you feel? b. Use specific emotion words like angry, sad, helpless, scared, hurt, hopeless, disappointed.	What do (did) you do or think about doing?	What are (were) the costs benefits of using the subst
I just got in another fight with my boyfriend right after getting some money from my parents.	I felt angry and depressed. I was thinking I just want to feel better and stop thinking about all the crap going on around me.	I called my friend Tammy and asked her to bring me some liquor.	(+) It made me feel good have the bottle. I don't kn I just like it. It took the edge off for a little while. (−) My boyfriend got piss off at me again, and we g in another fight. I felt ashamed and hopele

Those with poor insight might require a greater level of assistance with this step. Use a timeline, if necessary, to retrospectively track the actions that led to using the substance (e.g., "I was feeling bored"; "I called a friend to come over but he couldn't"; "I got drunk in my apartment alone"). Next, have the client describe the feelings and thoughts or ideas going through his or her mind at the time of the identified trigger situation. This step is important because it helps to determine what need the person was trying to meet by using substances. Continue to prompt if the client provides a vague response or has difficulty identifying specific thoughts and feelings.

In the third column clients will write what they ended up doing, or, if they are completing this in the moment they will write what they are thinking about doing (e.g., buy beer, call drug dealer, smoke a joint). After this they will list the positive and negative consequences of the substance-using behavior. This includes consideration of the drug effects (e.g., escape, euphoria, paranoia, physical illness) as well as the effects of participating in the event (e.g., peer-family response, criminal activity, putting housing in

HEALTHY ALTERNATIVE BEHAVIOR	POSITIVE AND NEGATIVE CONSEQUENCES	CURRENT THOUGHTS AFTER CONSIDERING CONSEQUENCES OF USE OR NONUSE
What would be a more healthy alternative behavior?	What are the costs and benefits of the alternative behavior?	
I guess I could have tried to find something fun to do like go see a movie. Sometimes I will take a hot bath with bubbles and just try to escape.	(+) I could have avoided another fight. I would feel better about myself. I would not feel guilty about using my parents' money. (–) Nothing I do seems to take the pain away like drugs.	Maybe I should try to find some new ways to cool off when I'm upset. This pattern seems to be a vicious cycle.

jeopardy). Next, the client will need help listing healthy alternative behaviors that would allow them to meet their needs identified in column 2. In the next column have them list the pros and cons of this alternative behavior. Finally, discuss with them their thoughts and feelings regarding the consequences of substance use. It may be necessary to help them navigate any hurdles that might prevent them from engaging in alternative behaviors. Also, if they are having difficulty committing to using alternative behaviors, use the motivation-enhancement strategies previously described.

· · ·

In preparation for Tina's discharge, the focus turned to relapse prevention. Tina was taught how to identify triggers and consider alternative actions to using substances through the thought change worksheet (table 9.1). She was provided with several blank copies and was encouraged to practice using the tool often upon discharge. Also, she was encouraged to begin attending AA and NA meetings as often as she can. She was provided a list of local meetings and was encouraged to pick one that was close to her for each day of the week. She voiced concern about attending meetings because she did not like the one she went to a couple of years ago and is less comfortable in a group setting. The therapist explained that she may need to shop around before finding one she is comfortable with, but she should give them a fair trial. The last issue that needed to be addressed was medication adherence. Tina had stopped using her antidepressant medication when she began increasing her alcohol use. It was explained to her that feeling down is one of her triggers, and the medication will be key in her effort to develop a drug-free lifestyle. Also, the various medication-adherence strategies were used to increase the likelihood that she will take her medications consistently. During her treatment Tina was encouraged to add the information she thought was most helpful to her crisis action plan, and by the time she was discharged she had a comprehensive plan for staying stable and avoiding relapse.

10

Important Treatment Considerations

VARIOUS ISSUES that need to be considered when conducting acute psychiatric treatment are discussed in this final chapter. First, aspects of providing help to clients with a borderline personality disorder (BPD), or borderline traits, are reviewed. Next, some of the unique cultural perspectives regarding mental health treatment, as well as individual differences in treatment needs among varying ethnic groups, are described. Finally, the ways in which religion and spirituality can be important coping resources for some clients are presented.

UNIQUE CHALLENGES ASSOCIATED WITH THE BORDERLINE PERSONALITY

Many books and treatment manuals single out the borderline personality as a condition that is challenging for mental health service providers. The authors typically provide suggestions for developing a healthy therapeutic alliance, establishing and maintaining appropriate boundaries, dealing with transference and countertransference, and handling the frequent and varied crises that often afflict clients with a borderline personality. It is no accident that this diagnosis receives so much individual attention; these clients typically have troubling histories and developmental issues and do indeed require a higher level of thoughtfulness, planning, patience, and compassion on the part of the clinician.

Meissner (1993:184) captures the challenge of treating individuals with a borderline personality by stating, "At all levels of the borderline spectrum they present special problems that challenge the limits of therapeutic capacity and resource in all therapists and often create difficult therapeutic impasses that can come close to exhausting any given therapist's capacity to manage." Richard Moskovitz is among the various authors who have provided guidance for working with this clinical population. In his book Lost in the Mirror: An Inside Look at Borderline Personality Disorder (2001), Moskovitz provides insightful descriptions of borderline behavior and corresponding advice for clinicians, family members, and individuals recovering from this condition. He encourages clinicians to define and maintain clear boundaries and to define clear limits of responsibility. He also suggests that clinicians should define realistic expectations early to avoid becoming codependent, to reduce the capacity for splitting, and to effectively manage issues of confidentiality. Moskovitz also warns against any form of exploitation, from sexual misconduct to being deceitful or manipulative, as this can retraumatize the client, reinforce issues related to trust, or cause a severe emotional reaction.

For those clients who are more neurotic or impulsive, it is important to provide structure and develop appropriate limits by controlling the time and space within which the therapeutic intervention takes place (Meissner, 1993). In other words, it will be advantageous to set up a specific protocol for contact and to determine what constitutes an emergency and nonemergency. It may also be helpful if the number of clinicians who have contact with the client remains small so that the distress resulting from the client's interpersonal difficulties is not compounded. It can be difficult to establish structure and consistency and to provide a comfortable therapeutic environment when the treatment comes in the form of a team. Teams typically comprise service providers who have differing personalities, styles, and training backgrounds; therefore it may be necessary either to assign one worker for those with a borderline diagnosis or to make an extra effort to interact with the client consistently.

It may also be difficult to get clients with a borderline personality to commit to and stay engaged in the treatment process. In one study among patients who were assessed at a psychiatric emergency room, those with a personality disorder were at least two times more likely to refuse any follow-up care (Bruffaerts, Sabbe, & Demyttenaere, 2005). Motivational interviewing strategies may be helpful in the effort to engage the individual in treatment. It may also be necessary to collaborate with the person's family or with trusted individuals in the community, such as other mental health professionals, to build trust or make necessary accommodations. It is not uncommon for individuals with borderline personality disorder either to feel that they do not need help or to believe that there is nothing that can help them. An individualized or person-centered approach is important so the client feels in control and so that the clinician can avoid making recommendations that the client deems unsatisfactory.

Unfortunately the assorted challenges that clients with disordered personalities present with cause mental health service providers to have negative attitudes toward them. Purves and Sand (2009) assessed the attitudes among mental health crisis and triage clinicians toward clients with personality disorders. Their study showed a greater overall percentage of negative attitudes than positive attitudes toward working with patients who have a personality disorder diagnosis. Although these emotions may be difficult to avoid, it is important to attempt to mask them when working with the client and to seek supervision or consultation to appropriately express frustrations and resolve negative attitudes.

Another issue related to the treatment of persons diagnosed with BPD is defensive practice. For various reasons, mental health professionals may be more likely to use a defensive, short-term focused intervention even if there are negative overall or long-term treatment consequences (Paris, 2008; Krawitz & Batcheler, 2006). In a pilot study conducted by Krawitz and Batcheler (2006), 85 percent of a group of nurses, psychologists, and psychiatrists working in various adult psychiatric treatment centers agreed with the statement that during the preceding year they had "taken a treatment approach that you feel is not likely to be in the client's best interest but protects you from medicolegal repercussions." Eighteen percent of these individuals reported practicing defensively twelve to fifty-two times, and another 18 percent reported doing this more than fifty-two times. To explain how defensive efforts to improve short-term risk may increase overall risk, Krawitz and Batcheler write:

> Defensive practice may result in overly custodial interventions such as prolonged acute hospitalization, lengthy one-to-one observation of the patient and frequent or lengthy use of mental health legislation. These overly

custodial interventions may unintentionally decrease the effectiveness of efforts to help patients solve the problems that precipitate their suicidality, decrease the effectiveness of efforts to teach patients how to increase their safety in their natural environment and decrease the effectiveness of treatment aimed at supporting patients' view of themselves as capable. (2006:320)

These authors encourage mental health service providers to adopt an alternative approach, claiming:

> Crises need to be survived and are also valuable opportunities for learning about and changing chronic patterns, including alternatives to suicide and self-harm as ways of dealing with distress. There needs to be a balance between creating an environment that protects against short-term suicide risk and an environment that promotes and enables longer-term change, thereby protecting against suicide in the long term. (321)

Although it is important to heed the warnings against being overly defensive, those who treat individuals with BPD should also be vigilant and careful to avoid overlooking legitimate crises. In a study that involved extensive interviews of 180 recent suicide attempters, individuals diagnosed with BPD had greater severity of overall psychopathology, depression, hopelessness, suicidal ideation, past suicide attempts, and impairment in social problem solving skills (Berk et al., 2007). These characteristics will likely need to be addressed to decrease long-term suicide risk. Others have also shown that suicidal behavior in clients along the borderline spectrum is more than just attention seeking (Paris, 2002; Soloff et al., 2000).

This brief review is intended to help clinicians avoid harmful practices and to encourage further reading and training around providing care to clients along the borderline spectrum. The information provided is not sufficient to replace formal training in the treatment of this population. It is recommended that service providers who work with individuals with borderline or other personality disorders engage in ongoing training, consultation, and supervision to maintain competency.

CULTURAL PERSPECTIVES ON MENTAL HEALTH TREATMENT

It is important to consider various cultural perspectives on mental illness and mental health treatment for a number of reasons. A solid understanding of cultural differences can affect a clinician's ability to communicate with a client about concerns in a meaningful way, engage and keep the client in treatment, select appropriate interventions, and avoid doing harm. According to Tsai and colleagues (2004:120), "Cultural variation (or the lack of cultural variation) in the occurrence and course of mental illness and in the presentation of psychiatric symptoms all have implications for treatment. Most importantly, they highlight aspects of psychotherapy and other psychiatric treatments that may require modification to be effective with different cultural groups." This section is not intended to be a comprehensive guide to multicultural psychology or counseling. It is an introduction to some of the cultural differences among minority groups and offers suggestions for approaching these individuals clinically.

Different cultures often perceive mental illness and psychiatric treatment in different ways. The ability to understand these differences and to respond appropriately by making special accommodations, using the appropriate language, and including certain people or activities may be essential for effective mental health care. When working with clients experiencing acute psychiatric illness, it is very important to be able to communicate effectively and to engage the client, and many times families, in the treatment process. Therefore, being aware of how clients from different cultures might perceive mental health professionals and understanding their preferences for treatment is crucial.

In the 1999 surgeon general's report on mental health, the first report emphasizing this aspect of a person's health, Dr. David Satcher stated, "A constellation of barriers deters ethnic and racial minority group members from seeking treatment, and if individual members of groups succeed in accessing services, their treatment may be inappropriate to meet their needs." If an individual from a minority group is seeking mental health treatment, it likely means he or she is experiencing significant distress or acute mental illness; otherwise the various barriers would have been a deterrence. It is important to communicate an understanding of these barriers and to work diligently to dispel preconceived notions about mental health care. For instance, clinicians can make an extra effort to accommodate language preferences and to communicate with family or community supports to gain a more culturally sensitive perspective of the client's needs.

Some of the barriers to effective treatment that are directly related to ethnic and cultural differences are not as obvious as others. For instance, the field of ethnopsychopharmacology investigates differences in the response to medication among different ethnic groups (Satcher, 1999). Both genetic and psychosocial factors contribute to differences in response to medication, and both physicians and clinicians meeting with clients should be aware of this research. In one study, Lin, Anderson, and Poland (1997) found that a large percentage of African Americans and Asians are slow metabolizers of several antipsychotic and antidepressant medications. This can affect the effectiveness of medications in managing symptoms as well as the frequency and severity of side effects.

Satcher later provided a summary of cultural issues in mental heath care in a supplement to his 1999 report, stating:

> The cultures from which people hail affect all aspects of mental health and illness, including the types of stresses they confront, whether they seek help, what types of help they seek, what symptoms and concerns they bring to clinical attention, and what types of coping styles and social supports they possess. Likewise, the cultures of clinicians and service systems influence the nature of mental health services. (U.S. Department of Health and Human Services, 2001)

Understandably, it will seem too daunting a task to develop a comprehensive knowledge base of all cultures; however, every bit of information about the varying cultural perspectives is important and can facilitate the provision of satisfactory treatment. To enhance cultural competence, some of the important treatment considerations that are unique to individuals from various selected minority groups are described in this section. Since there is often more diversity within various ethnic populations than between them, this information should not be used to reinforce stereotypes or create a rigid dichotomy of groups. Instead, clinicians should use this limited information as a starting place for engagement and inquiry in an effort to fully understand the individual seeking help.

First, some general suggestions should be made. It is recommended that clinicians refrain from being overly assumptive while attempting to be culturally sensitive and instead approach clients of different cultural backgrounds with accommodating flexibility and respectful curiosity. Also, as Das and Kemp (1997:32) have suggested, "Counselors and therapists need to keep in mind two key concepts, in addition to a general knowledge of cultural values: (a) the degree of acculturation that the client has undergone in the mainstream culture, and (b) the type of ethnic cultural identity that the client has developed." Additionally, some families will want to hide issues from people within the family; therefore it is necessary to ask about topics that can and cannot be discussed with everyone. Examples of questions to ask individuals or families to avoid problems related to cultural differences are as follows:

- What do you think about mental health treatment?
- Who do you want to be involved?
- How do you understand these problems?
- What do you believe would be helpful?
- What is your comfort with the English language?
- Who makes decisions in your home?

Arab American and Chaldean

As with many other ethnic groups, there is a stigma attached to mental illness within the Arabic and Chaldean cultures, and many less acculturated immigrants from the Middle East (e.g., Syria, Iraq, Egypt, Lebanon, Jordan, Palestine, Saudi Arabia) may circumvent mental health care to prevent the experience of shame (Hakim-Larson et al., 2007). According to Hakim-Larson and colleagues, acculturation issues and histories of trauma related to the immigration process and current political issues and world events are common culturally relevant concerns that mental health service providers are likely to see with Arab and Chaldean Americans. They also emphasize the need to understand the family unit because of the importance of culture and religion within family life. It is important to know that many Arab and Chaldean immigrants maintain collectivistic attitudes and perspectives, which may conflict with ideals found in Western mental health care practice (e.g., a strong focus on individual needs and developing personal autonomy). Also, men are traditionally acknowledged as heads of household.

During times of stress the extended family and religious group are traditionally seen as a support network for these ethnic groups (Hakim-Larson et al., 2007). However, families may be broken during immigration, or the support network in America may be limited or absent, causing this resource to be lacking. Another thing that can affect the family system is acculturation to the dominant culture. Mental health issues related to acculturation are typically more prevalent among Muslim Arab immigrants than among those with a Christian faith (Amer & Hovey, 2007; Amer, 2005). A study that assessed acculturative stress among Muslim Arab American families found that a longer length of residence in the United States was related to more life satisfaction but less family satisfaction (Faragallah, Schumm, and Webb, 1997). Furthermore, in a study that assessed socio-demographic differences in acculturation patterns among early immigrant and second-generation Arab Americans, religiosity was predictive of better family functioning and less depression within the Muslim population (Amer & Hovey, 2007).

It is also common for these ethnic groups to have a more external locus of control, meaning they attribute life events to fate or God's will (Nydell, 2006). This orientation toward the world may at times appear as a lack of motivation to change, and it may be used to absolve personal responsibility for past or future behavior. At the same time the belief that a higher power is in control can be comforting to the individual during times of distress. It is important to consult with culturally relevant persons in the community when helping Arab American clients and to focus on goals related to improving family relations and happiness rather than diagnostic labels or various problems (Amer, 2005). Arab Americans are also likely to prefer a brief intervention that is solution focused (Abudabbeh, 2005).

Jewish

Many Jewish individuals are comfortable with accessing mental health services. This is due in part to the fact that they are comfortable with being verbal and are knowledgeable about psychotherapy (Rosen & Weltman, 2005). The fact than there are many Jewish psychologists and psychiatrists may also be a factor. Clients who are Orthodox Jews, however, may have difficulty seeking out and participating fully in mental health treatment. According to Schnall (2006), there is concern that receiving mental health care will be seen as a sign of weakness. Some may also worry that mental health practitioners will ridicule their religious and community values, or they may be suspicious about psychotherapy and simply want to avoid participating in this aspect of secular society.

It may be helpful to provide assurance of confidentiality to Orthodox Jewish clients and to avoid involving family or friends in the treatment process. Many clients will prefer to receive services at a clinic outside their orthodox community (Feinberg & Feinberg, 1985). In some instances it may be appropriate to refrain from referring clients to support groups because of stigma concerns (Schnall, 2006). Mirkin and Okun (2005) have suggested that psychoeducation may be necessary to improve the client's understanding of psychological conditions.

African American and Black Caribbean

In a study that assessed mental health care usage and satisfaction among a large sample of African American and black Caribbean individuals in the United States, black Caribbean people who were third generation or later reported they were significantly less satisfied with mental health services received than did those who were first or second generation. Additionally, this group's reported satisfaction with mental health services was lower than the level of satisfaction reported by the African American respondents (Jackson et al., 2007). The third-generation group was also more likely to use mental health services. One of the possible explanations for the low level of satisfaction might be that black people of Caribbean descent seem to be more likely than white people to be referred by a nonhealth professional or be involuntarily detained (Morgan, et al., 2005; Oluwatayo & Gater, 2004). Knowledge of these findings might help clinicians to prepare for a client who may have negative attitudes about mental health care in America and to explore ways to make the experience more helpful.

Several researchers have analyzed data from the National Survey of Black Americans and found that most black Americans, including those who identify as African American, are likely to use informal resources during times of distress, and others will use a combination of informal and professional resources (Woodward, Taylor, & Chatters, 2011; Neighbors et al., 2007; Neighbors & Jackson, 1984). This seems to indicate a need to prepare informal sources for coping support (e.g., churches and community centers) to be able to effectively help individuals in their community. In other words, mental health professionals who are working with African American clients should assess their client's help-seeking patterns and if necessary help family members, pastors, extended family, and any others involved in the support network to be prepared to help in time of need. This might involve education, providing a list of community resources, instruction on crisis management strategies, and inclusion in the formal treatment that is being provided through hospital diversion or other services.

Researchers found that black Americans with emotional problems were less likely to seek help than those with other problems (e.g., physical problems). Additionally, older black individuals were more likely than younger individuals to seek no help at all (Woodward et al., 2010; Neighbors & Jackson, 1984). Barriers to help seeking may include low income, lack of transportation, and a limited support or social network. Hines and Boyd-Franklin (2005) suggest it is important to communicate respect, inquire into available family supports, and use a strengths-based approach when working with African Americans and their families.

A few research findings should be noted that specifically address the efficacy of mental health treatments with African American individuals. For instance, African Americans may not respond as well as whites to behavioral treatment for agoraphobia (Chambless & Williams, 1995) or exposure therapy for panic attacks (Williams & Chambless, 1994). Also, African Americans may metabolize some psychiatric medications, such as antidepressants and antipsychotics, more slowly than Whites (Bradford, Gaedigk, & Leeder, 1998; Ziegler & Biggs, 1977); thus lower doses should be prescribed to reduce negative side effects (Livingston et al., 1983). Treatments for PTSD and cognitive-behavioral treatment for anxiety have been shown to be equally effective among the two groups (Treadwell Flannery-Schroeder, & Kendall, 1995; Friedman, Paradis, & Hatch, 1994). Certainly there will be a range of responses to various treatments among African American clients, but the point here is that cultural factors should be considered along with motivational and other factors when developing treatment plans and explaining treatment outcomes.

Hispanic American

Persons of Mexican origin constitute the largest proportion of Hispanic Americans (nearly two-thirds). The remaining distribution includes primarily persons of Puerto Rican, Cuban, and Central American origin (U.S. Census Bureau, 2011). A combination of financial struggles, language barriers, discrimination, and other one-time and chronic issues have made life in the United States a struggle for many Hispanic Americans. These challenges also make it difficult to access necessary mental health services and other community resources (U.S. Department of Health and Human Services, 2001).

There are a number of culture-bound syndromes that Hispanic individuals might present within an acute-care setting. For instance, ataque de nervios (a condition most similar to panic attacks because it involves a sense of being out of control) can include symptoms such as shouting, crying, trembling, body warmth, verbal and physical aggression, and suicidal gestures. Also, the term locura refers to a condition of severe chronic psychosis and is characterized by symptoms typical of schizophrenia (American Psychiatric Association, 2000). Communication with the client and family members about the presenting problem and treatment plan might be aided by using these more familiar terms.

Mexican Americans are likely to respect authority, prioritize family unity, and value personalism (i.e., acknowledge unique personal qualities). They will likely prefer a treatment approach in which demands for disclosure are kept to a minimum, and they may have difficulty focusing on individual as opposed to family needs (Garcia-Preto, 2005). According to Garcia-Preto, the respect that Mexican Americans have for authority may cause them to avoid disagreeing with the clinician. It is important, then, to convey that it is safe and helpful to respond openly and honestly during the assessment and intervention process.

According to Zuniga (1997), Mexican American seniors may struggle with issues related to competence, autonomy, and relatedness. Feelings of incompetence and lack of autonomy are likely a result of difficulties stemming from not being able to speak English, limited education, and increased dependency on others. Evaluating the individual's system and facilitating changes in the way various persons interact, including the delineation of roles and provision of support, may be among the necessary clinical activities when providing care to this population. As with most seniors, it is important to not interact with older Mexican Americans in an overly patronizing manner. This may reinforce their feelings of incompetence and undermine the effort to increase confidence in social interactions, feelings of hopefulness, and a sense of personal worth and respect.

Many Hispanic families draw on their spirituality to cope with their own or a relative's serious mental illness (Guarnaccia et al., 1992). Also, research has demonstrated that Mexican American individuals with schizophrenia are less likely to relapse when they return to a family that is high in warmth and low in criticism (Lopez et al., 1999). Therefore, assisting the Mexican American client with maintaining stability will likely involve the encouragement of spiritual practices and inclusion of the family. As with many other minority groups, ethnic matching between clinician and client has been found to improve treatment participation and outcomes (Zane et al., 2005; Sue et al., 1991).

Asian American and South Asian American

Asian Americans have the lowest rate of mental health treatment utilization among the many ethnic populations (Lee & Mock, 2005). Shame and stigma related to mental illness, limited finances, differing conceptions of health and illness, and a shortage of culturally competent services are among the contributing factors (Lee & Mock, 2005; Sue & Sue, 1999). One of the reasons stigma is so pronounced is because in collectivist Asian cultures mental illness can reflect poorly on one's family lineage and negatively affect important aspects of social life, such as marriage opportunities (U.S. Dept. of Health and Human Services, 2001). Most Asian American groups value the ability to suppress outward expression of emotion and prefer not to dwell on upsetting thoughts (Wong et al., 2010; Parker, Cheah, & Roy, 2001; Kleinman, 1977; Tseng & Hsu, 1970).

Asian Americans are unlikely to seek mental health treatment unless all other efforts at achieving relief (e.g., spirituality alone or more holistic treatments) have failed. Characteristics of Asian Americans who are vulnerable to mental health problems may include female gender, older age, employment or financial difficulties, social isolation, and recent immigration. The resulting symptomatology is frequently depressive and/or somatic in nature (Lee & Mock, 2005).

Research has revealed a U-shaped curve when assessing the impact of immigration on mental health for individuals from various cultures. Asian populations are among the groups that experience an initial euphoria upon arriving to the United States but often begin to experience high levels of acculturative stress during the second and third years, followed by a decrease in stress as time goes by (Rumbaut, 1989; Ying, 1988; Hurh & Kim, 1988).

Being aware of this pattern might be helpful in determining triggers for the individual's current symptoms; therefore further inquiry is warranted if the client is a recent immigrant.

South Asian Americans include people from India, among others. There is great diversity in religious belief and practice in India (e.g., Hinduism, Islam, Christianity, Sikhism, Buddhism), and this aspect of the client's personal and social life should be considered when providing mental health treatment (Almeida, 2005; Das & Kemp, 1997). The various difficulties related to identity formation that are common to other cultures are also experienced among South Asian Americans. For instance, they may feel torn between adhering to traditional cultural norms, such as dress and behavior, and trying to blend in with the more dominant culture (Das & Kemp, 1997). The process of trying to develop a bicultural identity, or an identity that incorporates aspects of both dominant white and Indian cultures, can be challenging and a significant source of distress.

The inherent values related to individualism and autonomy found in traditional psychotherapy and counseling theory and practice may present problems when working with Asian American and South Asian Americans (Lee & Mock, 2005; Das & Kemp, 1997). Traditional values such as a strong sense of duty and strict obedience to the family and devaluation of individualism may make it difficult to trust mental health professionals who focus on individual needs. The bicultural tension that some already feel might be increased unintentionally because of these value differences. Das and Kemp (1997:31) have also noted that, for the South Asian American, "there is a cultural proscription against talking about personal, intimate problems with anyone other than a member of the family [and] people are reluctant to seek counseling because it will stigmatize not only the person who needs help, but also their entire family." These are some of the reasons why it is important to assess a person's level of acculturation.

The tendency of many Asian Americans to suppress affective expressions of distress often leads to somatization, or expression of physical symptoms (Karasz, Dempsey, & Falleck, 2007; Mak & Zane, 2004; Chun, Enomoto, & Sue, 1996; Nguyen, 1982; Kleinman, 1977). For instance, neurasthenia, which is a condition often characterized by fatigue, weakness, poor concentration, memory issues, irritability, aches and pains, and sleep disturbances, is a commonly diagnosed (ICD-10) condition in China (Yamamoto, 1992).

Koreans may experience hwa-byung, a culture-bound disorder with both somatic and psychological symptoms, such as pressure in the chest, palpitations, sensations of heat, flushing, headache, dysphoria, anxiety, irritability, and problems with concentration (Park, Kim, Schwartz-Barcott, & Kim, 2002; Prince, 1989; Lin, 1983). This could make the diagnosis of depression or anxiety according to the DSM-IV more complicated as the affective symptoms may not be endorsed, while physical symptoms will be emphasized. The clinical assessment needs to be thorough enough to determine if physical complaints are related to mental health issues or if a referral to a primary care physician is needed.

In sum, there are a number of differences in access to mental health treatment, views of mental illness, and treatment preferences among and within cultural groups. Providers of mental health care are responsible for maintaining a certain level of familiarity with these cultural differences. Also, clinicians have their own cultural biases and attitudes, and they must monitor their thoughts and feelings to ensure they do not pose a barrier to effective care. Finally, the key to culturally sensitive mental health care is to be proactive in learning about the individual client's unique needs and preferences and to accommodate them accordingly.

RELIGION AND SPIRITUALITY AS A COPING RESOURCE

In a study that assessed religious coping among 379 individuals with persistent mental illness, more than 81 percent of participants reported using religious beliefs or activities to cope. Furthermore, 65 percent perceived religion as effective, and the majority devoted up to 50 percent of their total coping time to religion (Rogers et al., 2002). In a similar study that involved 115 patients diagnosed with "schizophrenia or other nonaffective psychoses," 45 percent of patients reported that religion was the most important element in their lives, and 71 percent used religion as a positive way of coping (Huguelet, Mohr, & Borras, 2009). Several other studies further illustrate the common use of religion or spirituality to cope among individuals with mental illness (e.g., Mohr et al., 2006; Corrigan et al., 2003; Kirov et al., 1998).

These studies are unlikely to surprise mental health professionals who have worked with severely mentally ill individuals. It is quite common to witness or hear about the utilization of religious beliefs and activities (prayer, listening to religious music, attending services, reading religious texts, meditation) among these people. However, even though religious coping has been identified as an important factor in the recovery process for those with serious mental illness, mental health professionals may be doing little to acknowledge this and to incorporate religion into the treatment process (Hathaway, Scott, & Garver, 2004; Rogers et al., 2002). In a report of the UK's Mental Health Foundation titled *The Impact of Spirituality on Mental Health: A Review of the Literature*, Deborah Cornah (2006) states, "The key implication from the research is that the potential benefits of spiritual and religious expression and activity for mental health should not be overlooked by those in mental health services. However, for many, this is exactly what appears to happen."

In reference to providing family therapy to families of African origin, Black and Jackson (2002:81) claim that "a family's strong spiritual values may influence the meaning it assigns to a crisis and the options for resolution it considers. Clinician's understanding of these spiritual values is essential, both in terms of how a problem may challenge or threaten spiritual beliefs, and how spiritual values can be drawn on to resolve problems." This statement is likely relevant to clients and families of most cultural backgrounds, and it demonstrates how religion and spirituality can be intricately woven into the fabric of one's life. Cornah (2006) summarized this point well by stating, "Spirituality is a concept that evades simplistic definition, categorization or measurement and yet it affects the social, emotional, psychological and intellectual dimensions of our lives."

McLennan, Rochow, & Arthur (2001:136) illustrate further some of the potential benefits of considering the client's religious and spiritual beliefs and practices when providing counseling interventions: "Incorporating religious principles and practices such as forgiveness, prayer or meditation may be effective coping strategies for clients. Exploring or clarifying personal beliefs may provide them with a sense of purpose in life and meaning in suffering. Religious communities can be a rich source of practical, social, and emotional support."

There are many possibilities when it comes to adding a spiritual component to the treatment process. For example, clinicians have successfully incorporated Jewish ritual, such as prayer, into the treatment of various groups of Orthodox Jewish patients, including older people and those with psychosis (Witztum & Buchbinder, 2001; Heilman & Witztum, 2000;

Abromawitz, 1993; Bilu & Witztum, 1993). The key is to work with the client or family in understanding how religious and spiritual beliefs and practices might be relevant to the treatment process

For many people significant distress and hardship is the main thing that motivates them to turn to religion. They consider calling on a higher power only when they are between a rock and a hard place. It might be the case that people who experience serious mental illness engage in religious coping so often because they are continuously facing such circumstances. It is to be hoped that future research will shed light on this phenomenon, but for now clinicians need only be aware that religious coping is important to this clinical population and strive to facilitate the use of this resource when appropriate. Clinicians can start by assessing clients' preferences for using religion and spirituality at the beginning of the treatment process and then assisting them in restoring their religious and spiritual functioning in whatever ways possible, such as linking them to community groups, transporting them to services, or providing opportunities to discuss this aspect of their lives in therapy sessions.

CONCLUSION

People can recover from serious mental illness and lead fulfilling and productive lives. Those with serious mental health problems are no longer seen as people who simply need to be contained and secluded from society. Instead, more people are realizing that those with schizophrenia, bipolar disorder, and other illnesses can be great contributors to their communities. Success depends on their ability to reduce the strength and impact of various liabilities and to more effectively overcome acute symptom episodes. Mental health professionals play a key role in this process.

Those who are entrusted to provide acute mental health care take on a tremendous responsibility, and this work can be very challenging. The complicated issues that individuals experiencing severe mental illness often present with require a multimodal approach. The model outlined in this text is comprehensive. If followed it will help support clients on their road to recovery. When all spheres of a person's life become healthier, the occurrence and severity of acute symptom episodes will diminish. Furthermore, as support staff and clinicians become competent in using the various techniques discussed in this text, client hospitalizations will be reduced, the quality of client's lives will improve, and clinicians will be more satisfied with their work.

Thank you for being one of the large number of professionals who have committed to helping individuals with severe mental illness along their recovery journey. We hope that through reading this text you were able to add to your clinical toolbox and are left even more inspired to provide effective interventions each time you meet with those you serve.

Crisis Action Plan

SOME THINGS ABOUT ME

When I am feeling well, I am . . . (e.g., bright, cheerful, talkative, outgoing, active, energetic, humorous, a jokester, happy, dramatic, optimistic, curious, reasonable, responsible, industrious, supportive, calm, quiet, easy to get along with, argumentative, playful, withdrawn, introverted, extraverted, impulsive, friendly)

_____

_____

_____

_____

_____

_____

When I am feeling bad, I am . . . (e.g., depressed, anxious, feeling very sensitive or fragile, sleeping all the time, not sleeping, increased pain, having racing thoughts, having thoughts of self-harm, wanting to be alone, engaging in risk-taking behavior, spending a lot of money, taking anger out on others, seeing or hearing things that aren't really there, smoking a lot, feeling numb, blacking out or losing time, abusing substances, having suicidal thoughts, unable to concentrate)

_____
_____
_____
_____
_____
_____
_____

Stressors (things that may increase my symptoms or make me feel sad, angry, anxious, etc.) include . . . (e.g., being alone, financial problems, relationship problems, using alcohol/drugs, particular people, stopping my medication)

_____
_____
_____
_____
_____
_____
_____

Resources that are available to me for help during a crisis include . . . (e.g., people, places, community programs, churches, groups, clinics, activities)

_____
_____
_____
_____
_____
_____
_____

SOME THINGS OTHER PEOPLE CAN DO FOR ME

Specific things my counselor can do for me are . . . (include name, activity, time, other details)

_____
_____
_____

_____
_____
_____
_____

Specific things my family can do for me are . . .

_____
_____
_____
_____
_____
_____
_____

Specific things my doctor can do for me are . . .

_____
_____
_____
_____
_____
_____
_____

Specific things my friends can do for me are . . .

_____
_____
_____
_____
_____
_____
_____

SOME THINGS I NEED TO DO

To feel better and maintain my wellness, I need to do these specific things
each day (e.g., go for a walk, eat three healthy meals, get eight hours of sleep,
do thirty minutes of yoga, pray, bathe, avoid drugs/alcohol):

_____

_____

_____

_____

_____

_____

_____

To keep from getting ill or feeling worse when a triggering event occurs, I need to . . . (e.g., talk to a support, remember that it is okay to take care of myself, focus on tasks that are easy for me to do well, engage in prayer or some form of spiritual activity, get some exercise, write in my journal, do some deep-breathing or relaxation exercises, work on changing negative thoughts into positive)

Trigger: _____

Coping strategy: _____

Trigger: _____

Coping strategy: _____

Trigger: _____

Coping strategy: _____

Trigger: _____

Coping strategy: _____

NOTES

_____

_____

_____

_____

_____

_____

_____

_____

_____

OTHER INFORMATION

Name _____

Address _____

Personal telephone numbers _____

Psychiatric emergency number _____

Case manager _____

Therapist _____

Psychiatrist _____

Family _____

Employer _____

Insurance _____

Allergies _____

Medications _____

_____

_____

_____

_____

_____

Diagnosis (mental health) _____

_____

_____

_____

_____

_____

Diagnosis (physical health) _____

_____

_____

_____

_____

_____

Thought Change Worksheet

Thought Change Worksheet

1. SITUATION	2. RESPONSE	3. AUTOMATIC THOUGHT
Describe what is (was) going on at the time you experience(d) distress. Who? What? When? Where?	a. What do (did) you feel? b. Use specific words like *angry, sad, helpless, scared, hurt, hopeless, disappointed.*	a. What was going through your mind just before you started feel this way? Any Images? b. Circle the *trouble* thought (the one most connected to the distress).

The occurrence of frequent and related dysfunctional thoughts suggest a maladaptive schema, or ay of relating to the world, such as a *failure* or *self-sacrifice schema.*

Practice challenging past or present dysfunctional thoughts, and related schemas, *daily* to improve your emotional health and behavior.

VIDENCE THAT PORTS THE UBLE THOUGHT	5. EVIDENCE THAT DOES NOT SUPPORT THE TROUBLE THOUGHT	6. ALTERNATIVE / BALANCED THOUGHTS
:he *facts* that suggest the ɔle thought is *true*.	List the *facts* that suggest the trouble thought is *not true*.	a. Write an alternative or balanced thought considering the *facts*. b. Rate how much you believe in the alternative or balanced thought (1–10).

Thought Change Worksheet (Substance Abuse)

1. TRIGGER SITUATION	2. RESPONSE	3. SUBSTANCE USE BEHAVIOR	4. POSITIVE AND NEGATIVE CONSEQUENCES
Who? What? When? Where?	a. What do (did) you feel? b. What is (was) going through your mind? What thoughts do (did) you have?	What are (were) you thinking about using in response to the feelings and thoughts?	What are (were) the cost and benefits of using the substance?

Practice challenging past or present dysfunctional thoughts *daily* to prevent relapse and to develop healthy coping strategies..

5. HEALTHY ALTERNATIVE BEHAVIOR	6. POSITIVE AND NEGATIVE CONSEQUENCES	7. CURRENT THOUGHTS AFTER CONSIDERING CONSEQUENCES OF USE VS. NONUSE
What would be a more healthy alternative behavior?	What are the costs and benefits of the alternative behavior?	

Stress-Vulnerability Model Diagrams

JAR =
Capacity for stress before
psychotic break/relapse

BALL =
Various acute and
chronic stressors

GOAL =
Decrease stressors,
create space in order to
resolve/prevent crisis
[i.e., hallucinations,
aggression, anxiety,
depression, suicidal
behavior]

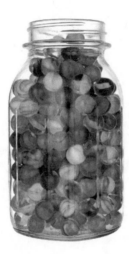

FIGURE C.1 Vulnerability Stress-Jar Metaphor

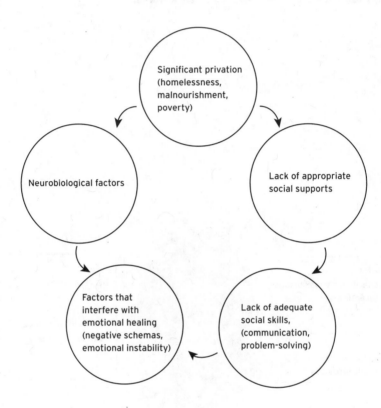

FIGURE C.2 Psychological Liabilities

REFERENCES

Abramowitz, L. (1993). Prayer as therapy among the frail Jewish elderly. *Journal of Gerontological Social Work, 19*(3/4), 69–75.

Abudabbeh, N. (2005). Arab families: An overview. In M. McGoldrick, J. Giordano, & N. Garcia-Preto (Eds.), *Ethnicity and Family Therapy* (3rd ed., pp. 423–36). New York: Guilford.

Alexander, P. E. (1991). Management of panic disorders. *Journal of Psychoactive Drugs, 23*(4), 329–33.

Almeida, R. (2005). Asian Indian families: An overview. In M. McGoldrick, J. Giordano, & N. Garcia-Preto (Eds.), *Ethnicity and Family Therapy* (3rd ed., pp. 377–94). New York: Guilford.

Amer, M. M. (2005). Arab American mental health in the Post September 11 era: Acculturation, stress, and coping. *Dissertation Abstracts International: Section B: The Sciences and Engineering, 66*(4-B), 1974.

Amer, M. M., & Hovey, J. D. (2007). Socio-demographic differences in acculturation and mental health for a sample of 2nd generation/early immigrant Arab Americans. *Journal of Immigrant and Minority Health, 9*(4), 335–47.

American Psychiatric Association. (1994). Practice guidelines for the treatment of patients with bipolar disorder. *American Journal of Psychiatry, 151* (Suppl. 12).

———. (2000). *Diagnostic and statistical manual of mental disorders* (4th ed., text rev.). Washington, D.C.: Author.

Anchin, J. C. (2003). Cybernetic systems, existential phenomenology, and solution-focused narrative: Therapeutic transformation of negative affective states through integratively oriented brief psychotherapy. *Journal of Psychotherapy Integration, 13*, 334–442.

———. (2008). Contextualizing discourse on a philosophy of science for psychotherapy integration. *Journal of Psychotherapy Integration, 18*(1), 1–24.

Anderson, R. C., & Grunert, B. K. (1997). A cognitive behavioral approach to the treatment of post-traumatic stress disorder after work-related trauma. *Professional Safety, 42*(11), 39–43.

Antonuccio, D. O. (1998). The coping with depression course: A behavioral treatment for depression. *Clinical Psychologist, 51*, 3–5.

Antonuccio, D. O., Lewinsohn, P., Piasecki, M., & Ferguson, R. (2000). Major depressive episode. In M. Hersen & M. Biaggio (Eds.), *Effective brief therapies: A clinician's guide* (pp. 19–40). San Diego: Academic.

Attkisson, C., Cook, J., Karno, M., Lehman, A., McGlashan, T. H., Meltzer, H. Y., O'Connor, M., Richardson, D., Rosenblatt, A., Wells, K., Williams, J., & Hohmann, A. A. (1992). Clinical services research. *Schizophrenia Bulletin, 18*, 561–626.

Audini, B., Marks, I. M., Lawrence R. E., Connolly, T., & Watts, V. (1994). Home-based versus outpatient/inpatient care for people with serious mental illness: Phase II of a controlled study. *British Journal of Psychiatry, 165*, 179–94.

Baker, A., Lee, N. K., Claire, M., Lewin, T. J., Grant, T., Pohlman, S., et al. (2005). Brief cognitive behavioural interventions for regular amphetamine users: A step in the right direction. *Addiction, 100*(3), 367–78.

Baker, A., Lewin, T., Reichler, H., Clancy, R., Carr, V., Garrett, R., et al. (2002). Evaluation of a motivational interview for substance use within psychiatric inpatient services. *Addiction, 97*(10), 1329.

Baker, J. A. (2000). Developing psychosocial care for acute psychiatric wards. *Journal of Psychiatric & Mental Health Nursing, 7*(2), 95.

Bakker, A., Van Balkom, A., & Spinhoven, P. (2002). SSRIs vs. TCAs in the treatment of panic disorder: A meta-analysis. *Acta Psychiatrica Scandanavica, 106*, 163–67.

Baldessarini, R. J., Tondo, L., Hennen, J., & Viguera, A. C. (2002). Is lithium still worth using? An update of selected recent research. *Harvard Review of Psychiatry, 10*(2), 59.

Ball, J., Mitchell, P., Malhi, G., Skillecorn, A., & Smith, M. (2003). Schema-focused cognitive therapy for bipolar disorder: Reducing vulnerability to relapse through attitudinal change. *Australian and New Zealand Journal of Psychiatry, 37*(1), 41–48.

Ball, J. S., Links, P. S., Strike, C., & Boydell, K. M. (2005). "It's overwhelming ... everything seems to be too much": A theory of crisis for individuals with severe and persistent mental illness. *Psychiatric Rehabilitation Journal, 29*(1), 10–17.

Ball, S. A., Martino, S., Nich, C., Frankforter, T. L., Van Horn, D., Crits-Christoph, P., et al. (2007). Site matters: Multisite randomized trial of motivational enhancement therapy in community drug abuse clinics. *Journal of Consulting and Clinical Psychology, 75*(4), 556–67.

Barlow, D. H. (2009, March). A unified protocol for the treatment and prevention of emotional disorders. Paper presented as part of the Regent University colloquium series, Virginia Beach.

Barlow, D. H., Craske, M. G., Cerny, J. A., & Klosko, J. S. (1989). Behavioral treatment of panic disorder. *Behavior Therapy, 20*, 429–57.

Barlow, D. H., Gorman, J. M., Shear, M. K., & Woods, S. W. (2000). Cognitive-behavioral therapy, imipramine, or their combination for panic disorder: A randomized controlled trial. *Journal of the American Medical Association, 283*, 2529–36.

Barlow, J. H., Ellard, D. R., Hainsworth, J. M., Jones, F. R. & Fisher, A. (2005). A review of self-management interventions for panic disorders, phobias and obsessive-compulsive disorders. *Acta Psychiatrica Scandinavica, 111*, 272–85.

Barrowclough, C., Haddock, G., Tarrier, N., Lewis, S. W., Moring, J., O'Brien, R., et al. (2001). Randomized controlled trial of motivational interviewing, cognitive behavior therapy, and family intervention for patients with comorbid schizophrenia and substance use disorders. *American Journal of Psychiatry, 158*(10), 1706–13.

Beamish, P. M., Granello, D. H., & Belcastro, A. L. (2002). Treatment of panic disorder: Practical Guidelines. *Journal of Mental Health Counseling, 24*(3), 224–46.

Beamish, P. M., Granello, P. F., Granello, D. H., McSteen, P. B., Bender, B. A., & Hermon, D. (1996). Outcome studies in the treatment of panic disorder: A review. *Journal of Counseling & Development, 74*, 460–67.

Bechdolf, A., Klosterkötter, J., Hambrecht, M., Knost, B., Kuntermann, C., Schiller, S., et al. (2003). Determinants of subjective quality of life in post acute patients with schizophrenia. *European Archives of Psychiatry & Clinical Neuroscience, 253*(5), 228–35.

Bechdolf, A., Köhn, B., Knost, B., Pukrop, R., & Klosterkötter, J. (2005). A randomized comparison of group cognitive-behavioural therapy and group psychoeducation in acute patients with schizophrenia: Outcome at 24 months. *Acta Psychiatrica Scandinavica, 112*(3), 173–79.

Beck, A. T., Sokol, L., Clark, D. A., Berchick, R., & Wright, F. (1992). A crossover study of focused cognitive therapy for panic disorder. *American Journal of Psychiatry, 149*, 778–83.

Bellino, S., Zizza, M., Rinaldi, C., & Bogetto, F. (2007). Combined therapy of major depression with concomitant borderline personality disorder: Comparison of interpersonal and cognitive psychotherapy. *Canadian Journal of Psychiatry, 52*(11), 718–25.

Ben-Porath, D. D., Peterson, G., & Piskur, C. (2004). Effectiveness of and consumer satisfaction with an assertive community treatment program for the severely mentally ill: A 3-year follow-up. *Psychological Services, 1*(1), 40–47.

Berk, M. S., Jeglic, E., Brown, G. K., Henriques, G. R., & Beck, A. T. (2007). Characteristics of recent suicide attempters with and without borderline personality disorder. *Archives of Suicide Research, 11*, 91–104.

Bernstein, J., Bernstein, E., Tassiopoulos, K., Heeren, T., Levenson, S., & Hingson, R. (2005). Brief motivational intervention at a clinic visit reduces cocaine and heroin use. *Drug Alcohol Depend, 77*(1), 49–59.

Beutler, L. E. (1983). *Eclectic psychotherapy: A systematic approach*. Elmsford, N.Y.: Pergamon.

Beutler, L. E., & Clarkin, J. (1990). *Systematic treatment selection: Toward targeted therapeutic interventions*. New York: Brunner/Mazel.

Beutler, L. E., Clarkin, J., & Bongar, B. (2000). *Guidelines for the systematic treatment of the depressed patient*. New York: Brunner/Mazel.

Beutler, L. E., Consoli, A., & Lane, G. (2005). Systematic treatment selection and prescriptive psychotherapy: An integrative eclectic approach. In J. Norcross & M. Goldfried (Eds.), *Handbook of psychotherapy integration* (2nd ed., pp. 121–46). New York: Oxford University Press.

Beutler, L. E., Engle, D., Mohr, D., Daldrup, R. J., Bergan, J., Meredith, K., & Merry, W. (1991). Predictors of differential response to cognitive, experiential and self-directed psychotherapeutic procedures. *Journal of Consulting and Clinical Psychology, 59*, 333–40.

Beutler, L. E., Goodrich, G., Fisher, D., & Williams, R. E. (1999). Use of psychological tests/instruments for treatment planning. In M. Maruish (Ed.), *Use of psychological testing for treatment planning and outcome assessment* (2nd ed., pp. 81–113). Hillsdale, N.J.: Lawrence Erlbaum.

Beutler, L. E., & Harwood, M. (2000). *Prescriptive psychotherapy: A practical guide to systematic treatment selection*. New York: Oxford University Press.

Beutler, L. E., & Mitchell, R. (1981). Differential psychotherapy outcome among depressed and impulsive patients as a function of analytic and experiential treatment procedures. *Psychiatry, 44*, 297–306.

Beutler, L. E., Mohr, D.C., Grawe, K., Engle, D., & MacDonald, R. (1991). Looking for differential treatment effects: Cross-cultural predictors of differential psychotherapy efficacy. *Journal of Psychotherapy Integration, 1*, 121–41.

Beutler, L. E., Moleiro, C., Malik, M., Harwood, T. M., Romanelli, R., Gallagher-Thompson, D., et al., (2003). A comparison of the dodo, EST, and ATI indicators among co-morbid stimulant dependent, depressed patients. *Clinical Psychology & Psychotherapy, 10*, 69–85.

Bilu, Y., & Witztum, E. (1993). Working with Jewish Ultra-Orthodox patients: Guidelines for a culturally sensitive therapy. *Culture, Medicine and Psychiatry, 17*(2), 197–233.

Black, D. W., Wesner, R., Bowers, W., & Gabel, J. (1993). A comparison of fluvoxamine, cognitive therapy, and placebo in the treatment of panic disorder. *Archives of General Psychiatry, 50*, 44–50.

Black, L., & Jackson, V. (2005). Families of African origin: An overview. In M. McGoldrick, J. Giordano, & N. Garcia-Preto (Eds.), *Ethnicity and Family Therapy* (3rd ed., pp. 77–86). New York: Guilford.

Blow, F. C., Ullman, E., Lawton Barry, K., Bingham, C. R., Copeland, L. A., McCormick, R., et al. (2000). Effectiveness of specialized treatment programs for veterans with serious and persistent mental illness: A three-year follow-up. *American Journal of Orthopsychiatry, 70*(3), 389–400.

Blume, A. W., & Marlatt, G. A. (2009). The role of executive cognitive functions in changing substance use: What we know and what we need to know. *Annals of Behavioral Medicine, 37*, 117–25.

Bond, G. R., Drake, R. E., Mueser, K. T., & Latimer, E. (2001). Assertive community treatment for people with severe mental illness: Critical ingredients and impact on patients. *Disease Management & Health Outcomes, 9*(3), 141–59.

Bonsack, C., Adam, L., Haefliger, T., Besson, J., & Conus, P. (2005). Difficult-to-engage patients: A specific target for time-limited assertive outreach in a Swiss setting. *The Canadian Journal of Psychiatry / La Revue Canadienne De Psychiatrie, 50*(13), 845–50.

Bradford, L. D., Gaedigk, A., & Leeder, J. S. (1998). High frequency of CYP2D6 poor and "intermediate" metabolizers in black populations: A review and preliminary data. *Psychopharmacology Bulletin, 34*, 797–804.

Brendel, D. H. (2003). Reductionism, integrativeism, and pragmatism in psychiatry: The dialectic of clinical explanation. *Journal of Medicine and Philosophy, 28*(5–6), 563–80.

Brown, G. K., Beck, A. T., Steer, R. A., & Grisham, J. R. (2000). Risk factors for suicide in psychiatric outpatients: A 20-year prospective study. *Journal of Consulting and Clinical Psychology, 68*, 371–77.

Bruchner, T. A., & Yoon, J. (2009). Does deinstitutionalization increase suicide? *Health Services Research, 44*, 1385+.

Bruffaerts, R., Sabbe, M., & Demyttenaere, K. (2005). Predicting aftercare in psychiatric emergencies. *Social Psychiatry & Psychiatric Epidemiology, 40,* 829–34.

Callahan, J. (1994). Defining crisis and emergency. *Crisis: The Journal of Crisis Intervention and Suicide Prevention, 15*(4), 164–71.

Calvert, S. J., Beutler, L. E., & Crago, M. (1988). Psychotherapy outcome as a function of therapist-patient matching on selected variables. *Journal of Social and Clinical Psychology, 6,* 104–17.

Cauce, A.M., Hannan, K., & Sargeant. (1992). Life stress, social support, and locus of control during early adolescence: interactive effects. *American Journal of Community Psychology, 20,* 787–99.

Chadwick, P., Birchwood, M., & Trower, P. (1996). *Cognitive therapy for delusions, voices, and paranoia.* West Sussex: Wiley.

Chambless, D. L., & Williams, K. E. (1995). A preliminary study of the effects of exposure in vivo for African Americans with agoraphobia. *Behavior Therapy, 26,* 501–15.

Chinman, M., Allende, M., Bailey, P., Maust, J., & Davidson, L. (1999). Therapeutic agents of assertive community treatment. *Psychiatric Quarterly, 70*(2), 137–62.

Chun, C., Enomoto, K., & Sue, S. (1996). Health care issues among Asian Americans: Implications of somatization. In P. M. Kato & T. Mann (Eds.), *Handbook of diversity issues in health psychology* (pp. 347–66). New York: Plenum.

Clum, G. A., Clum, G. A., & Surls, R. (1993). A meta-analysis of treatment for panic disorder. *Journal of Consulting and Clinical Psychology, 61,* 317–26.

Cochran, S. D. (1984). Preventing medical noncompliance in the outpatient treatment of bipolar affective disorder. *Journal of Consulting and Clinical Psychology, 52*(5), 873–78.

Colom, F., & Vieta, E. (2004). A perspective on the use of psychoeducation, cognitive-behavioral therapy and interpersonal therapy for bipolar patients. *Bipolar Disorders, 6*(6), 480–86.

Colom, F., Vieta, E., Sanchez-Moreno, J., Martínez-Arán, A., Torrent, C., Reinares, M., et al. (2004). Psychoeducation in bipolar patients with comorbid personality disorders. *Bipolar Disorders, 6*(4), 294–98.

Commonwealth of Virginia Office of the Governor Press Office. (2001, January 8). *Governor Gilmore announces historic mental health restructuring plan.* http://www.lva.lib.va.us/archives/gilmore/press/news2001/menheo108.htm.

Copeland, M. E. (2007). *Mental health recovery including wellness recovery action Planning.* http://mentalhealthrecovery.com/art_wrap.php.

Cornah, D. (2006). *The impact of spirituality on mental health: A review of the literature.* http://www.bacip.org.uk/_fileuploads/mh+foundation+spirituality+report.pdf.

Corrigan P., McCorkle B., Schell B., et al. (2003). Religion and spirituality in the lives of people with serious mental illness. *Community Mental Health Journal, 39,* 487–99.

Corrigan, P., & Ralph, R. (2005). Introduction: Recovery as consumer vision and research paradigm. In R. Ralph & P. Corrigan (Eds.), *Recovery in mental illness: Broadening our understanding of wellness* (pp. 3–17). Washington, D.C.: American Psychological Association.

Craddock, N., & Forty, L. (2006). Genetics of affective (mood) disorders. *European Journal of Human Genetics, 14*(6), 660–68.

Craske, M. G., & Barlow, D. H. (2001). Panic disorder and agoraphobia. In D. Barlow (Ed.), *Clinical handbook of psychological disorders: A step-by-step treatment manual* (3rd ed., pp. 1–59). New York: Guilford.

Craske, M. G., Brown, T. A., & Barlow, D. H. (1991). Behavioral treatment of panic disorder: A two year follow up. *Behavior Therapy, 22,* 289–304.

Das, A., & Kemp, S. (1997). Between Two Worlds: Counseling South Asian Americans. *Journal of Multicultural Counseling & Development, 25*(1), 23–33.

Datillio, F. (2001). Crisis intervention techniques for panic disorder. *American Journal of Psychotherapy, 55*(3), 388–405.

DeRubeis, R. J., Gelfand, L. A., Tang, T. Z., & Simons, A. D. (1999). Medications versus cognitive behavior therapy for severely depressed outpatients: Mega-analysis of four randomized comparisons. *American Journal of Psychiatry, 156*(7), 1007–13.

DiClemente, C. C., & Velasquez, M. M. (2002). Motivational interviewing and the stages of change. In W. R. Miller, & S. Rollnick (Eds.), *Motivational Interviewing: Preparing people for change* (2nd ed., pp. 201–16). New York: Guilford.

Doane, J. A., Goldstein, M. J., Miklowitz, D. J., & Falloon, I. R. (1986). The impact of individual and family treatment on the affective climate of families of schizophrenics. *British Journal of Psychiatry, 148,* 279–87.

Drake, R. E., McHugo, G. J., Clark, R. E., Teague, G. B., Xie, H., Miles, K., et al. (1998). Assertive community treatment for patients with co-occurring severe mental illness and substance use disorder: A clinical trial. *American Journal of Orthopsychiatry, 68*(2), 201–15.

Drury, V., Birchwood, M., Cochrane, R., & MacMillan, F. (1996a). Cognitive therapy and recovery from acute psychosis: A controlled trial: I. Impact on psychotic symptoms. *British Journal of Psychiatry, 169*, 593–601.

———. (1996b). Cognitive therapy and recovery from acute psychosis: A controlled trial: II. Impact on recovery time. *British Journal of Psychiatry, 169*, 601–7.

Dunn, C., DeRoo, L., & Rivara, F. P. (2001). The use of brief interventions adapted from motivational interviewing across behavioral domains: A systematic review. *Addiction, 96*(12), 1725–42.

Eagle, G. T. (1998). An integrative model for brief term intervention in the treatment of psychological trauma. *International Journal of Psychotherapy, 3*(2), 135–47.

Eells, T. D. (2000). Psychotherapy of schizophrenia. *Journal of Psychotherapy Practice and Research, 9*(4): 250–54.

Elkin, I., Gibbons, R. D., Shea, M. T., Sotsky, S. M., Watkins, J. T., Pilkonis, P. A., et al. (1995). Initial severity and differential treatment outcome in the national institute of mental health treatment of depression collaborative research program. *Journal of Consulting and Clinical Psychology, 63*(5), 841–47.

Elkin, I., Shea, M. T, Watkins, J. T, Imber, S. D., Sotsky, S. M., Collins, J. E, Glass, D. R., Pilkonis, P. A., Leber, W R., Docherty, J. P., Fiester, S. J., & Parloff, M. B. (1989). NIMH Treatment of Depression Collaborative Research Program: General effectiveness of treatments. *Archives of General Psychiatry, 46*, 971–83.

Elliott, C., & Smith, L. (2003). *Overcoming anxiety for dummies.* New York: Wiley.

Essock, S. M., Frisman, L. K., & Kontos, N. J. (1998). Cost-effectiveness of assertive community treatment teams. *American Journal of Orthopsychiatry, 68*(2), 179–90.

Evans, L., Holt, C., & Oei, T. P. S. (1991). Long term follow-up of agoraphobics treated by brief intensive group cognitive behavior therapy. *Australian and New Zealand Journal of Psychiatry, 25*, 343–49.

Ewing, J. A. (1984). Detecting Alcoholism: The CAGE Questionnaire. *JAMA, 252*(14), 1905–7.

Fagiolini, A., Kupfer, D. J., Rucci, P., Scott, J. A., Novick, D. M., & Frank, E. (2004). Suicide attempts and ideation in patients with bipolar I disorder. *Journal of Clinical Psychiatry, 65*(4), 509–14.

Fahy, T. J., O'Rourke, D., Brophy, J., et al. (1992). The Galway study of panic disorder I. Clomiprimine and lofeprimine in DSM-III-R panic disorder: A placebo-controlled trial. *Journal of Affective Disorders, 25*, 63–76.

Falloon, I. R. H. (2002). Cognitive-behavioral family and educational interventions for schizophrenic disorders. In S. Hofmann & M. Tompson (Eds.), *Treating chronic and severe mental disorders: A handbook of empirically supported interventions* (pp. 3–17). New York: Guilford.

Falloon, I. R. H., Barbieri, L., Boggian, I., & Lamonaca, D. (2007). Problem solving training for schizophrenia: Rationale and review. *Journal of Mental Health*, *16*(5), 553–68.

Falloon, I. R. H., Held, T., Coverdale, J. H., Roncone, R., & Laidlaw, T. M. (1999). Family interventions for schizophrenia: A review of long-term benefits of international studies. *Psychiatric Rehabilitation Skills*, *3*(2), 268–90.

Faragallah, M. H., Schumm, H. R., & Webb, F. J. (1997). Acculturation of Arab American immigrants: An exploratory study. *Journal of Comparative Family Studies*, *28*, 182–203.

Feinberg, S. & Feinberg, K. (1985). An assessment of the mental health needs of the Orthodox Jewish population of Metropolitan New York. *Conference of Jewish Communal Service*, *62*(1), 29–39.

Fenton, W. S. (2000). Evolving perspectives on individual psychotherapy for schizophrenia. *Schizophrenia Bulletin*, *26*(1), 47–72.

First, M. B., & Tasman, A. (2005). DSM-IV-TR Mental Disorders: Diagnosis, Etiology, & Treatment. West Sussex: Wiley.

Fisher, D., Beutler, L. E., & Williams, O. B. (1999). Making assessment relevant to treatment planning: The STS clinician rating form. *Journal of Clinical Psychology*, *55*, 825–42.

Foa, E. B., Hearst-Ikeda, D., & Perry, K. J. (1995). Evaluation of a brief cognitive-behavioral program for the prevention of chronic PTSD in recent assault victims. *Journal of Consulting and Clinical Psychology*, *63*, 948–55.

Foa, E. B., Rothbaum, B. O., Riggs, D. S., & Murdock, T. B. (1991). Treatment of posttraumatic stress disorder in rape victims: A comparison between cognitive-behavioral procedures and counseling. *Journal of Consulting and Clinical Psychology*, *59*, 715–23.

Forbes, D., Creamer, M., Phelps, A., Bryant, R., McFarlane, A., Devilly, G., Matthews, L., Raphael, B., Doran, C., Merlin, T., & Newton, S. (2007). Australian guidelines for the treatment of adults with acute stress disorder and posttraumatic stress disorder. *Australian and New Zealand Journal of Psychiatry*, *41*, 637–48.

Fosha, D. (2004). Brief integrative therapy comes of age: A commentary. *Journal of Psychotherapy Integration*, *14*(1), 66–92.

Frank, E., Anderson, B., Stewart, B. D., Dancu, C. Hughes, C., & West, D. (1988). Efficacy of cognitive behavior therapy and systematic desensitization in the treatment of rape trauma. *Behavior Therapy, 19,* 403–20.

Frank, E., Kupfer, D. J., Thase, M. E., Mallinger, A. G., Swartz, H. A., Fagiolini, A.M., et al. (2005). Two-year outcomes for interpersonal and social rhythm therapy in individuals with bipolar I disorder. *Archives of General Psychiatry, 62*(9), 996–1004.

Frank, E., Soreca, I., Swartz, H. A., Fagiolini, A.M., Mallinger, A. G., Thase, M. E., et al. (2008). The role of interpersonal and social rhythm therapy in improving occupational functioning in patients with bipolar I disorder. *American Journal of Psychiatry, 165*(12), 1559–65.

Frank, E., Swartz, H. A., & Kupfer, D. J. (2000). Interpersonal and social rhythm therapy: Managing the chaos of bipolar disorder. *Biological Psychiatry, 48*(6), 593–604.

Frankl, V. (2006). *Man's Search for Meaning.* Boston: Beacon.

Friedman, S., Paradis, C. M., & Hatch, M. (1994). Characteristics of African-American and white patients with panic disorder and agoraphobia. *Hospital and Community Psychiatry, 45,* 798–803.

Friedmann, C., & Silvers, F. (1977). A multimodality approach to inpatient treatment of obsessive-compulsive disorder. *American Journal of Psychotherapy, 31*(3), 456–66.

Fyer, A. J., Liebowitz, M. R., Gorman, J. M., & Campeas, R. (1987). Discontinuation of alprazolam treatment in panic patients. *American Journal of Psychiatry, 144*(3), 303–8.

Garcia-Preto, N. (2005). Latino families: An overview. In M. McGoldrick, J. Giordano, & N. Garcia-Preto (Eds.), *Ethnicity and Family Therapy* (3rd ed., pp. 153–65). New York: Guilford.

Garssen, B., de Ruiter, C., & van Dyck. (1992). Breathing retraining: A rational placebo? *Clinical Psychology Review, 12,* 141–53.

Gersons, B., Carlier, I., Lamberts, R., & van der Kolk, B. (2000). Randomized clinical trial of brief integrative psychotherapy for police officers with posttraumatic stress disorder. *Journal of Traumatic Stress, 13*(2) 333–47.

Gitlin, M. J., Swendsen, J., Heller, T. L., & Hammen, C. (1995). Relapse and impairment in bipolar disorder. *American Journal of Psychiatry, 152*(11), 1635–40.

Gloagen, V., Cottraux, J., Cucherat, M., & Blackburn, I. M. (1998). A meta-analysis of the effects of cognitive therapy in depressed patients. *Journal of Affective Disorders, 49,* 59–72.

Goldberg, J. F., & Truman, C. J. (2003). Antidepressant-induced mania: An overview of current controversies. *Bipolar Disorders, 5*(6), 407–20.

Goldfried, M. R., Pachankis, J. E., & Bell, A. C. (2005). A history of psychotherapy integration. In J. Norcross & M. Goldfried (Eds.), *Handbook of psychotherapy integration* (2nd ed., pp. 24–60). New York: Oxford University Press.

Goldman, R. N., Greenberg, L. S., & Angus, L. (2006). The effects of adding emotion-focused interventions to the client-centered relationship conditions in the treatment of depression. *Psychotherapy Research, 16*(5), 536–46.

Gonda, X., Fountoulakis, K. N., Kaprinis, G., & Rihmer, Z. (2007). Prediction and prevention of suicide in patients with unipolar depression and anxiety. *Annals of General Psychiatry, 6*, 23–28.

Granello, D., Granello, P., & Lee, F. (1999). Measuring treatment outcomes and client satisfaction in a partial hospitalization program. *Journal of Behavioral Health Services and Research, 26*(1), 50–63.

Grawe, R., Falloon, I., Widen, J. & Skogvoll, E. (2006). Two years of continued early treatment for recent-onset schizophrenia: A randomised controlled study. *Acta Psychiatrica Scandinavica, 114*, 328–36.

Grech, E. (2002). Psychological interventions for psychosis: A critical review of the current evidence. *Internet Journal of Mental Health, 1*(2), 23.

Grob, G. N. (2008, Sept. 18). Mental health policy in 20th century America. In SAMHSA'S National Mental Health Information Center, *Section 1: Looking ahead and reflecting upon the past.* http://mentalhealth.samhsa.gov/publications/allpubs/SMA01-3537/chapter2.asp.

Guarnaccia, P. J., Parra, P., Deschamps, A., Milstein, G., & Argiles, N. (1992). Si Dios quiere: Hispanic families' experiences of caring for a seriously mentally ill family member. *Culture, Medicine and Psychiatry, 16*, 187–215.

Hacker Hughes, J., & Thompson, J. (1994). Post traumatic stress disorder: An evaluation of behavioural and cognitive behavioural interventions and treatments. *Clinical Psychology and Psychotherapy, 1*(3), 125–42.

Haddock, G., Barrowclough, C., Tarrier, N., Moring, J., O'Brien, R., Schofield, N., et al. (2003). Cognitive-behavioural therapy and motivational intervention for schizophrenia and substance misuse: 18-month outcomes of a randomised controlled trial. *British Journal of Psychiatry, 183*(5), 418–26.

Haddock, G., Tarrier, N., Morrison, A. P., Hopkins, R., Drake, R., & Lewis, S. (1999). A pilot study evaluating the effectiveness of individual inpatient cognitive-behavioral therapy in early psychosis. *Social Psychiatry and Psychiatric Epidemiology, 34*, 254–58.

Hakim-Larson, J., Kamoo, R., Nassar-McMillan, S. C., & Porcerelli, J. H. (2007). Counseling Arab and Chaldean American families. *Journal of Mental Health Counseling, 29*(4), 301–21.

Haringsma, R., Engels G., Van Der Leeden, R. & Spinhoven, P. (2006). Predictors of response to the "Coping with Depression" course for older adults: A field study. *Aging & Mental Health, 10*(4) 424–34.

Harvard Mental Health Letter. (1996). Post-traumatic stress disorder-part II. *Harvard Mental Health Letter, 13*(1), 1–6.

Hathaway, W. L., Scott, S. Y., & Garver, S. A. (2004). Assessing religious/spiritual functioning: A neglected domain in clinical practice. *Professional Psychology: Research and Practice, 35*(1), 97–104.

Heath, D. S. (2005). *Home treatment for acute mental disorders: An alternative to hospitalization.* New York: Routledge.

Hegerl, U., Plattner, A., & Möller, H.-J. (2003). Should combined pharmaco- and psychotherapy be offered to depressed patients? A qualitative review of randomized clinical trials from the 1990s. *European Archives of Psychiatry Clinical Neuroscience, 254*, 99–107.

Heilman, S. C., & Witztum, E. (2000). All in faith: Religion as the idiom and means of coping with distress. *Mental Health, Religion & Culture, 3*(2), 115–24.

Heinssen, R. K., Liberman, R. P., & Kopelowicz, A. (2000). Psychosocial skills training for schizophrenia: Lessons from the laboratory. *Schizophrenia Bulletin, 26*(1), 21–46.

Herman, J. L. (1992). *Trauma and recovery.* New York: Basic Books.

Himmelhoch, J. M., Fuchs, C. Z., May, S. J., Symons, B. J., & Neil, J. F. (1981). When a schizoaffective diagnosis has meaning. *Journal of Nervous and Mental Disease, 169*(5), 277–82.

Hines, P. M., & Boyd-Franklin, N. (2005). African American families. In M. Mc-Goldrick, J. Giordano, & N. Garcia-Preto (Eds.), *Ethnicity and Family Therapy* (3rd ed., pp. 87–100). New York: Guilford.

Hocking, C., Phare, J., & Wilson, J. (2005). Everyday life following long term psychiatric hospitalisation. *Health Sociology Review, 14*(3), 297.

Hofmann, S., & Tompson, M. (Eds.). (2002). *Treating chronic and severe mental disorders: A handbook of empirically supported interventions.* New York: Guilford.

Hogarty, G. E. (2002). Personal therapy: A practical psychotherapy for the stabilization of schizophrenia. In S. Hofmann & M. Tompson (Eds.), *Treating chronic and severe mental disorders: A handbook of empirically supported interventions* (pp. 53–68). New York: Guilford.

Hogarty, G. E., Anderson, C. M., Reiss, D. J., & Kornblith, S. J. (1991). Family psychoeducation, social skills training, and maintenance chemotherapy in the aftercare treatment of schizophrenia. II. Two-year effects of a controlled study on relapse and adjustment. *Archives of General Psychiatry, 48*(4), 340–47.

Hogarty, G. E., Anderson, C. M., Reiss, D. J., Kornblith, S. J., Greenwald, D. P., Javna, C. D., et al. (1986). Family psychoeducation, social skills training, and maintenance chemotherapy in the aftercare treatment of schizophrenia. I. One-year effects of a controlled study on relapse and expressed emotion. *Archives of General Psychiatry, 43*(7), 633–42.

Hogarty, G. E., Kornblith, S. J., Greenwald, D., DiBarry, A. L., Cooley, S., Ulrich, R. F., et al. (1997). Three-year trials of personal therapy among schizophrenic patients living with or independent of family: I. Description of study and effects of relapse rates. *American Journal of Psychiatry, 154*(11), 1504–13.

Huguelet, P., Mohr, S., & Borras, L. (2009). Recovery, spirituality, and religiousness in schizophrenia. *Clinical Schizophrenia & Related Psychoses, 2*(4), 307–16.

Human Services of New Mexico (2008). Assertive community treatment (ACT) services. *New Mexico Human Services Register, 31*(4), 6.

Hunter, S., Paddock, S. Ebener, P., Burkhart, A. K., & Chinman, M. (2009). Promoting evidence-based practices: The adoption of a prevention support system in community settings. *Journal of Community Psychology, 37*(5), 579–93.

Hurh, W. M., & Kim, K. C. (1988). *Uprooting and adjustment: A sociological study of Korean immigrants' mental health (Final report to the National Institute of Mental Health).* Macomb: Western Illinois University, Department of Sociology and Anthropology.

Husted, J., & Wentler, S. (2000). The effectiveness of day treatment with persistently mentally ill in rural areas. *Disability and Rehabilitation, 22*(9), 423–26.

Huxley, N. A., Parikh, S. V., & Baldessarini, R. J. (2000). Effectiveness of psychosocial treatments in bipolar disorder: State of the evidence. *Harvard Review of Psychiatry, 8*(3), 126–40.

Jackson, J. S., Neighbors, H. W., Torres, M., Martin, L. A., & Williams, D. R. (2007). Use of mental health services and subjective satisfaction with treatment among Black Caribbean immigrants: Results from the National Survey of American Life. *American Journal of Public Health, 97*(1), 60–67.

James, R. K., & Gilliland, B. E. (2001). *Crisis intervention strategies* (4th ed.). Belmont, Calif.: Wadsworth.

Jerrell, J. M. (1999). Skill, symptom, and satisfaction changes in three service models for people with psychiatric disability. *Psychiatric Rehabilitation Journal*, 22(4), 342.

Joiner, T. (2005). *Why people die by suicide*. Cambridge: Harvard University Press

Kahler, C. W., Read, J. P., Ramsey, S. E., Stuart, G. L., McCrady, B. S., & Brown, R. A. (2004). Motivational enhancement for 12-step involvement among patients undergoing alcohol detoxification. *Journal of Consulting & Clinical Psychology*, 72(4), 736–41.

Kahn, R. J., McNair, D. M., & Lipman, R. S. (1986). Imiprimine and chlordiazepoxide in depressive and anxiety disorders: II. Efficacy in anxious outpatients. *Archives of General Psychiatry*, 43, 79–85.

Kaliski, S. Z. (1997). Risk management during the transition from hospital to community care. *International Review of Psychiatry*, 9(2), 249–56.

Kamis-Gould, E. Snyder, F. Hadley, T. & Casey, T. (1999). The impact of closing a state psychiatric hospital on the county mental health system and its clients. Psychiatric Services, 50(10), 1297–1302.

Kane, J. M. (1997). Update on treatment strategies. *International Review of Psychiatry*, 9(4), 419–28.

Kane, J. M., & McGlashan, T. H. (1995). Treatment of schizophrenia. *Lancet*, 346(8978), 820.

Karasz, A., Dempsey, K., & Fallek, R. (2007). Cultural differences in the experience of everyday symptoms: A comparative study of South Asian and European American Women. *Culture, Medicine & Psychiatry*, 31, 473–97.

Kay-Lambkin, F., Baker, A., & Lewin, T. (2004). The "co-morbidity roundabout": A framework to guide assessment and intervention strategies and engineer change among people with co-morbid problems. *Drug & Alcohol Review*, 23(4), 407–23.

Keane, T. M., Street, A. E., & Orcutt, H. K. (2000). Posttraumatic stress disorder. In M. Hersen & M. Biaggio (Eds.), *Effective Brief Therapies: A Clinician's Guide* (pp. 139–55). San Diego: Academic Press.

Keck, P. E., McElroy, S. L., Strakowski, S. M., West, S. A., Sax, K. W., Hawkins, J. M., Bourne, M. L., & Haggard, P. (1998). 12-month outcome of patients with bipolar disorder following hospitalization for a manic or mixed episode. *American Journal of Psychiatry*, 155, 646–52.

Kelly, K., Rizvi, S., Monson, C. & Resick, P. (2009). The impact of sudden gains in cognitive behavioral therapy for posttraumatic stress disorder. *Journal of Traumatic Stress*, 22(4), 287–93.

Kerr, I. (2001). Brief cognitive analytic therapy for post-acute manic psychosis on a psychiatric intensive care unit. Clinical Psychology and Psychotherapy, 8, 117–29.

Kessler, R. C., Chiu, W. T., Demler, O., & Walters, E., E. (2005). Prevalence, severity, and comorbidity of 12-month DSM-IV disorders in the national comorbidity survey replication. Archives of General Psychiatry, 62(6), 617–27.

Kessler, R. C., Heeringa, S., Lakoma, M. D., Petukhova, M., Rupp, A. E., Schoenbaum, M., Wang, P. S., Zaslavsky, A.M. (2008). The individual-level and societal-level effects of mental disorders on earnings in the United States: Results from the National Comorbidity Survey Replication. American Journal of Psychiatry, published online ahead of print May 7, 2008.

Kevan, I., Gumley, A., & Coletta, V. (2007). Post-traumatic stress disorder in a person with a diagnosis of schizophrenia: Examining the efficacy of psychological intervention using single N methodology. Clinical Psychology and Psychotherapy, 14, 229–43.

Kingdon, D. G., & Turkington, D. (2005). Cognitive therapy of schizophrenia. New York: Guilford.

Kirov G., Kemp R., Kirov K., et al. (1998). Religious faith after psychotic illness. Psychopathology, 31, 234–45.

Kleinman, A. (1977). Depression, somatization and the "new cross-cultural psychiatry." Social Science and Medicine, 11, 3–10.

Klosko, J. S., Barlow, D. H., Tassinari, R., & Cerny, J. A. (1990). A comparison of alprazolam and behavior therapy in the treatment of panic disorder. Journal of Consulting and Clinical Psychology, 58, 77–84.

Knack, W. A. (2009). Psychotherapy and alcoholics anonymous: An integrated approach. Journal of Psychotherapy Integration, 19(1), 86–109.

Kobasa, S. C. (1979). Stressful life events, personality, and health: An inquiry into hardiness. Personality and Social Psychology, 37(1), 1–11.

Kohlenberg, R. J., Kanter, J., Bolling, M., Parker, C., & Tsai, M. (2002). Enhancing cognitive therapy for depression with Functional Analytic Psychotherapy: Treatment guidelines and empirical findings. Cognitive and Behavioral Practice, 9, 213–29.

Krawitz, R., & Batcheler, M. (2006). Borderline personality disorder: A pilot survey about clinician views on defensive practice. Australasian Psychiatry, 14(3), 320–22.

Krüger, S., Young, T. L., & Bräunig, P. (2005). Pharmacotherapy of bipolar mixed states. Bipolar Disorders, 7(3), 205–15.

Kuyken, W., Daigleish, T., & Holden, E. R. (2007). Advances in cognitive-behavioural therapy for umpolar depression. *Canadian Journal of Psychiatry, 52*(1), 5–13.

Kwee, M. (1984). *Klinische multimodale gedragstherapie.* Lisse, Holland: Swets & Zeitlinger.

Kwee, M., & Kwee-Taams, M. (1994). *Klinishegedragstherapie in Nederland & vlaanderen.* Delft, Holland: Eubron.

Lam, D. H., Bright, J., Jones, S., Hayward, P., Schuck, N., Chisholm, D., & Sham, P. (2000). Cognitive therapy for bipolar illness: A pilot study of relapse prevention. *Cognitive Therapy & Research, 24*(5), 503–21.

Lamb, R. (2001). Deinstitutionalization at the beginning of the new millennium. In R. Lamb & L. Weinberger (Eds.), *Deinstitutionalization: Promise and problems.* New York: Wiley.

Lampropoulos,G. (2000). Evolving psychotherapy integration: Eclectic selection and prescriptive applications of common factors in therapy. *Psychotherapy, 37*(4), 285–97.

Lancashire, S., Haddock, G., Tarrier, N., & Baguley, I. (1997). Effects of training in psychosocial interventions for community psychiatric nurses in England. *Psychiatric Services, 48*(1), 39–41.

Landau, J., Garrett, J., Shea, R., Stanton, M. D., Brinkman-Sull, D., & Baciewicz, G. (2000). Strength in numbers: The ARISE method for mobilizing family and network to engage substance abusers in treatment. *American Journal of Drug & Alcohol Abuse, 26*(3), 379–98.

Lang, E., Engelander, M., & Brooke, T. (2000, September). Report of an integrated brief intervention with self-defined problem cannabis users. *Journal of Substance Abuse Treatment, 19*(2), 111–16.

Latimer, E. (1999). Economic impacts of assertive community treatment: A review of the literature. *Canadian Journal of Psychiatry, 44*(5), 443–54.

———. (2005). Economic considerations associated with assertive community treatment and supported employment for people with severe mental illness. *Journal of Psychiatry & Neuroscience, 30*(5), 355–59.

Latimer, E., Bond, G., & Drake, R. (2011). Economic approaches to improving access to evidence-based and recovery-oriented services for people with severe mental illness. *Canadian Journal of Psychiatry, 56*(9), 523–29.

Lawson, D. M. (1995). Conceptualization and treatment for Vietnam veterans experiencing posttraumatic stress disorder. *Journal of Mental Health Counseling, 17*, 31–53.

Lazarus, A. (1981). *The practice of multimodal therapy.* New York: McGraw-Hill.

———. (1986). Multimodal therapy. In J. C. Norcross (Ed.). *Handbook of eclectic psychotherapy* (pp. 65–93). New York: Brummer/Mazel.

———. (1989). *The practice of multimodal therapy (Update).* Baltimore: Johns Hopkins University Press.

———.(1995). Different types of eclecticism and integration: Let's be aware of the dangers. *Journal of Psychotherapy Integration, 5* (1), 27–39.

———. (1997). *Brief but comprehensive psychotherapy: The multimodal way.* New York: Springer.

———. (2000). Multimodal therapy. In R. J. Corsini, & D. Wedding (Eds.), *Current psychotherapy* (6th ed). Itasca, Ill.: Peacock.

———. A. (2005a). Multimodal therapy. In J. Norcross & M. Goldfried (Eds.), *Handbook of psychotherapy integration* (2nd ed., pp. 105–20). New York: Oxford University Press.

———. (2005b). Is there still a need for psychotherapy integration? *Current Psychology, 24*(3), 149–52.

Lee, E., & Mock, M. R. (2005). Asian families: An overview. In M. McGoldrick, J. Giordano, & N. Garcia-Preto (Eds.), *Ethnicity and Family Therapy* (3rd ed., pp. 269–289). New York: Guilford.

Levenson, H. (2003). Time-limited dynamic psychotherapy: An integrationist perspective. *Journal of Psychotherapy Integration, 13,* 300–333.

Lewinsohn, P.M., Antonuccio, D. O., Steinmetz-Breckenridge, J. L., & Teri, L. (1984). *The coping with depression course: A psychoeducational intervention for unipolar depression.* Eugene, Ore.: Castalia.

Lewis, S., Tarrier, N., Haddock, G., Bentall, R., Kinderman, P., Kingdon, D., et al. (2002). Randomised controlled trial of cognitive-behavioural therapy in early schizophrenia: Acute-phase outcomes. *British Journal of Psychiatry, 181,* s91–s97.

Ligon, J., & Thyer, B. A. (2000). Client and family satisfaction with brief community mental health, substance abuse, and mobile crisis services in an urban setting. *Stress, Trauma, and Crisis: An International Journal, 6*(2), 93–99.

Lin, K. M., Anderson, D., & Poland, R. E. (1997). Ethnic and cultural considerations in psychopharmacotherapy. In D. Dunner (Ed.), *Current psychiatric therapy II* (pp. 75–81). Philadelphia: W. B. Saunders.

Lindauer, R., Gersons, B., van Meijel, E., Blom, K., Carlier, I., Vrijlandt. I, & Olff, M. (2005). Effects of brief integrative psychotherapy in patients with posttraumatic stress disorder: Randomized clinical trial. *Journal of Traumatic Stress, 18*(3), 205–12.

Linehan, M. (1993a). *Cognitive-behavioral treatment of borderline personality disorder.* New York: Guilford.

———. (1993b). *Skills training manual for treating borderline personality disorder.* New York: Guilford.

Links, P. S., Eynan, R., Ball, J. S., Barr, A., & Rourke, S. (2005). Crisis occurrence and resolution in patients with severe and persistent mental illness: The contribution of suicidality. *Crisis: The Journal of Crisis Intervention and Suicide Prevention, 26*(4), 160–69.

Lipton, L. (2001). Few safeguards govern elimination of psychiatric beds. *Psychiatric News, 36*(15), 9–29.

Livanou, M. (2001). Psychological treatments for post-traumatic stress disorder: An overview. *International Review of Psychiatry, 13*(3), 181–88.

Livingston, R. L., Zucker, D. K., Isenberg, K., & Wetzel, R. D. (1983). Tricyclic antidepressants and delirium. *Journal of Clinical Psychiatry, 44,* 173–76.

Lopez, S. R., Nelson, K. A., Snyder, K. S., & Mintz, J. (1999). Attributions and affective reactions of family members and course of schizophrenia. *Journal of Abnormal Psychology, 108,* 307–14.

Ma, S. H., & Teasdale, J. D. (2004). Mindfulness-based cognitive therapy for depression: Replication and exploration of differential relapse prevention effects. *Journal of Consulting and Clinical Psychology, 72,* 31–40.

Magnavita, J. J., & Carlson, T. M. (2003). Short-term restructuring psychotherapy: An integrative model for the personality disorders. *Journal of Psychotherapy Integration, 13,* 264–99.

Maisto, S. A., Carey, M. P., Carey, K. B., Gordon, C. M., & Gleason, J. R. (2000). Use of the AUDIT and the DAST-10 to identify alcohol and drug use disorders among adults with a severe and persistent mental illness. *Psychological Assessment, 12*(2), 186–92.

Mak, W. W. S., & Zane, N. W. S. (2004). The phenomenon of somatization among community Chinese Americans. *Social Psychiatry & Psychiatric Epidemiology, 39,* 967–74.

Malm, U., Ivarsson, B., Allebeck, P., & Falloon, I. R. H. (2003). Integrated care in schizophrenia: A 2-year randomized controlled study of two community-based treatment programs. *Acta Psychiatrica Scandinavica, 107*(6), 415.

Margraf, J., Barlow, D. H., Clark, D. M., & Telch, M. J. (1993). Psychological treatment of panic: Work in progress on outcome, active ingredients, and follow-up. *Behaviour Research and Therapy, 31,* 1–8.

Marlatt, G. A., and Gordon, J. R., eds. (1985). *Relapse Prevention: Maintenance Strategies in the Treatment of Addictive Behaviors.* New York: Guilford.

Maslow, A. H. (1970). *Motivation and personality* (2nd ed.). New York: Harper & Row.

Mastroeni, A., Bellotti, C., Pellegrini, E., Galletti, F., Lai, E., & Falloon, I. R. H. (2005). Clinical and social outcomes five years after closing a mental hospital: a trial of cognitive behavioural interventions. *Clinical Practice & Epidemological Mental Health, 23,* 1–25.

Matsakis, A. (1994). *Post-traumatic stress disorder: A complete treatment guide* (L. Tilley, Ed.). Oakland: New Harbinger.

McBride, T. D., Calsyn, R. J., Morse, G. A., Klinkenberg, W. D., & Allen, G. A. (1998). Duration of homeless spells among severely mentally ill individuals: A survival analysis. *Journal of Community Psychology, 26*(5), 473–90.

McCormack, N. A. (1985). Cognitive therapy of posttraumatic stress disorder: A case report. *American Mental Health Counselors Association Journal, 7,* 151–55.

McCracken, S. G., & Corrigan, P. W. (2008). Motivational interviewing for medication adherence in individuals with schizophrenia. In H. Arkowitz, H. A. Westra, W. R. Miller, & S. Rollnick (Eds.), *Motivational interviewing in the treatment of psychological problems* (pp. 249–76). New York: Guilford.

McCullough, J. P. (2003). Treatment for chronic depression: Cognitive behavioral analysis system of psychotherapy (CBASP). *Journal of Psychotherapy Integration, 13,* 241–63.

McKay, M., Fanning, P., & Paleg, K. (1994). *Couple skills: Making your relationship work.* Oakland: New Harbinger.

McKay, M., & Rogers, P. (2000). *The anger control workbook.* Oakland: New Harbinger.

McLennan, N., Rochow, S., & Arthur, N. (2001). Religious and Spiritual Diversity in Counselling. *Guidance & Counseling, 16*(4), 132–37.

McMinn, M., & Campbell, C. (2007). *Integrative psychotherapy: Toward a comprehensive Christian approach.* Downers Grove, Ill.: InterVarsity Press.

Mehrabian, A. (2001). General relations among drug use, alcohol use, and major indexes of psychopathology. *Journal of Psychology, 135*(1), 71–87.

Meichenbaum, D. (1974). *Cognitive behavior modification.* Morristown, N.J.: General Learning Press.

Meissner, W. W. (1993). Treatment of patients in the borderline spectrum: An overview. *American Journal of Psychotherapy, 47*(2), 184–93.

Menikoff, A. (1999a). *Psychiatric home care: Clinical and economic dimensions*. San Diego: Academic Press.

———. (1999b). The goals and principles of psychiatric home care. In A. Menikoff (Ed.), *Psychiatric home care: Clinical and economic dimensions* (pp. 39–57). San Diego: Academic.

Merson, S., Tryer, P., Onyett, S., Lack, S., Birkett, P., Lynch, S., & Johnson, T. (1992). Early intervention in psychiatric emergencies: A controlled trial. *Lancet, 339* (8805) 1311–15.

Messer, S. B. (1992). A critical examination of belief structures in integrative and eclectic psychotherapy. In J. C. Norcross & M. R. Goldfried (Eds.), *Handbook of psychotherapy integration* (pp. 130–65). New York: Basic Books.

Meuret, A. E., Wilhelm, F. H., & Roth, W. T. (2004). Respiratory feedback for treating panic disorder. *Journal of Clinical Psychology/In Session, 60*, 197–207.

Miklowitz, D. J. (2001). Bipolar disorder. In D. Barlow (Ed.), *Clinical handbook of psychological disorders: A step-by-step treatment manual* (3rd ed., pp. 523–61). New York: Guilford.

———. (2002). Family-focused treatment for bipolar disorder. In S. Hofmann & M. Tompson (Eds.), *Treating chronic and severe mental disorders: A handbook of empirically supported interventions* (pp. 159–74). New York: Guilford.

Miklowitz, D. J., George, E. L., Richards, J. A., Simoneau, T. L., & Suddath, R. L. (2003). A randomized study of family-focused psychoeducation and pharmacotherapy in the outpatient management of bipolar disorder. *Archives of General Psychiatry, 60*, 904–12.

Miklowitz, D. J., Goldstein, M. J., Nuechterlein, K. H., Snyder, K. S., & Mintz, J. (1988). Family factors and the course of bipolar affective disorder. *Archives of General Psychiatry, 45*, 225–31.

Miklowitz, D. J., Simoneau, T. L., George, E. A., Richards, J. A., Kalbag, A., Sachs-Ericsson, N., et al. (2000). Family-focused treatment of bipolar disorder: One-year effects of a psychoeducational program in conjunction with pharmacotherapy. *Biological Psychiatry, 48*, 582–92.

Miller, R. & Mason, S. E. (1999). Phase-specific psychosocial interventions for first-episode schizophrenia. *Bulletin of the Menninger Clinic, 63*(4), 499–519.

———. (2004). Cognitive enhancement therapy: A therapeutic treatment strategy for first-episode schizophrenic patients. *Bulletin of the Menninger Clinic, 68*(3), 213–30.

Miller, S., Duncan, B. L., & Hubble, M. A. (2005). Outcome-informed clinical work. In J. Norcross & M. Goldfried (Eds.), *Handbook of psychotherapy integration* (2nd ed., pp. 84–102). New York: Oxford University Press.

Miller, W. R., & DePilato, M. (1983). Treatment of nightmares via relaxation and desensitization: A controlled evaluation. *Journal of Consulting and Clinical Psychology, 51*, 870–77.

Miller, W. R. & Rollnick, S. (2002). *Motivational interviewing: Preparing people for change* (2nd ed.) New York: Guilford.

Miller, W. R., Yahne, C. E. & Tonigan, J. S. (2003). Motivational interviewing in drug abuse services: A randomized trial. *Journal of Consulting and Clinical Psychology, 71*, 754–63.

Min, M. O., Biegel, D. E., Johnsen, J. A. (2005). Predictors of psychiatric hospitalization for adults with co-occurring substance and mental disorders as compared to adults with mental illness only. *Psychiatric Rehabilitation Journal, 29*(2), 114–21.

Mirkin, M. P., & Okun, B. F. (2005). Orthodox Jewish families. In M. McGoldrick, J. Giordano, & N. Garcia-Preto (Eds.), *Ethnicity and Family Therapy* (3rd ed., pp. 689–700). New York: Guilford.

Mitchell, P. B. (2004). Australian and New Zealand clinical practice guidelines for the treatment of bipolar disorder. *Australian & New Zealand Journal of Psychiatry, 38*(5), 280–305.

Mohr S., Brandt P., Borras L., et al. (2006). Toward an integration of spirituality and religiousness into the psychosocial dimension of schizophrenia. *American Journal of Psychiatry, 163*, 1952–59.

Monti, P. M., Barnett, N. P., Colby, S. M., Gwaltney, C. J., Spirito, A., Rohsenow, D. J., et al. (2007). Motivational interviewing versus feedback only in emergency care for young adult problem drinking. *Addiction, 102*(8), 1234–43.

Monti, P. M., Rohsenow, D. J., Michalec, E., Martin, R. A., & Abrams, D. B. (1997). Brief coping skills treatment for cocaine abuse: Substance use outcomes at three months. *Addiction, 92*(12), 1717–28.

Morgan, C., Mallett, R., Hutchinson, G., Morgan, K., Dazzan P., McKenzie, K. et al. (2005). Pathways to care and ethnicity 2: Sources of referral and help-seeking. *British Journal of Psychiatry, 186*(4), 290–96.

Morris, C. D., Miklowitz, D. J., & Waxmonsky, J. A. (2007). Family-focused treatment for bipolar disorder in adults and youth. *Journal of Clinical Psychology, 63*(5; 5), 433–45.

Morrison, K. (1997). Personality correlates of the Five-Factor Model for a sample of business owners/managers: Associations with scores on *self*-monitoring, type A behavior, locus of control and subjective well-being. *Psychological Reports, 80* (1), 255–72.

Moses, E. B., & Barlow, D. H. (2006). A new unified treatment approach for emotional disorders based on emotion science. *Current Directions in Psychological Science, 15*(3), 146–50.

Moskovitz, R. (2001). *Lost in the mirror: An inside look at borderline personality disorder* (2nd ed.). Lanham, Md.: Taylor Trade.

Moyer, A., & Finney, J. W. (2004). Brief interventions for alcohol problems. *Alcohol Research & Health, 28*(1), 44–50.

Mueser, K. T. (2004). Clinical interventions for severe mental illness and co-occurring substance use disorder. *Acta Neuropsychiatrica, 16*(1), 26–35.

Mulder, R. (1982). *Final evaluation of the Harbinger Program as a demonstration project.* Lansing: Michigan Department of Mental Health.

Nadiga, D. N., Hensley, P. L., & Uhlenhuth, E. H. (2003). Review of the long-term effectiveness of cognitive behavioral therapy compared to medications in panic disorder. *Depression and Anxiety, 17,* 58–64.

National Institute for Clinical Excellence (NICE). (2005). *The management of PTSD in adults and children in primary and secondary care.* Wiltshire, U.K.: Cromwell Press.

National Institute of Mental Health (NIMH). (n.d.) *The Numbers Count: Mental Disorders in America.* http://www.nimh.nih.gov/health/publications/the-numbers-count-mental-disorders-in-america.shtml.

———. (1987). *Towards a model for a comprehensive community-based mental health system.* Washington, D.C.: NIMH.

Neighbors, H. W., Caldwell C., Williams, D. R., et al. (2007). Race, ethnicity, and the use of services for mental disorders: Results from the National Survey of American Life. *Archives of General Psychiatry, 64,* 485–94.

Neighbors, H. W., & Jackson, J. S. (1984). The use of informal and formal help: Four patterns of illness behavior in the black community. *American Journal of Community Psychology, 12*(6), 629–44.

Newman, M. G., Castonguay, L. G., & Borkovec, T. D. (June, 2002). Integrating cognitive-behavioral and interpersonal/emotional processing treatments for generalized anxiety disorder: Preliminary outcome findings. Paper presented at the Society for Psychotherapy Research, Santa Barbara, Calif.

Nguyen, S. D. (1982). Psychiatric and psychosomatic problems among Southeast Asian refugees. *Psychiatric Journal of the University of Ottawa, 7*, 163–72.

Nishith, P., Hearst, D. E., Mueser, K. T., & Foa, E. B. (1995). PTSD and major depression: Methodological and treatment considerations in a single case design. *Behavior Therapy, 26*, 319–35.

Norcross, J. C., Hedges, M., & Castle, P. H. (2002). Psychologists conducting psychotherapy in 2001: A study of the Division 29 membership. *Psychotherapy: Theory, Research, Practice, Training, 39*, 97–102.

North Carolina Department of Health and Human Services Division of Mental Health, Developmental Disabilities, and Substance Abuse Services. (2005). Communication bulletin #048—Transition plan for mobile crisis management.

Noyes, R., Caudry, D., & Domingo, D. (1986). Pharmacologic treatment of phobic disorders. *Journal of Clinical Psychiatry, 47*, 445–52.

Nydell, M. K. (2006). *Understanding Arabs: A guide for modern times* (4th ed.). Boston: Intercultural Press.

O'Connor, R. (2003). An integrative approach to treatment of depression. *Journal of Psychotherapy Integration, 13*(2), 130–70.

Oluwatayo, O., & Gater, R. (2004). The role of engagement with services in compulsory admission of African/Caribbean patients. *Social Psychiatry and Psychiatric Epidemiology, 39*(9), 739–43.

Otto, M. W., & Reilly-Harrington, N. (2002). Cognitive-behavioral therapy for the management of bipolar disorder. In S. Hofmann & M. Tompson (Eds.), *Treating chronic and severe mental disorders: A handbook of empirically supported interventions* (pp. 116–30). New York: Guilford.

Otto, M. W., Tolin, D. F., Nations, K. R., Utschig, A. C., Rothbaum, B. O. Hofmann, S. G., & Smits, J. (2012). Five sessions and counting: Considering ultra brief treatment for panic disorder. *Depression and Anxiety, 29*, 465–70.

Parabiaghi, A., Bonetto, C., Ruggeri, M., Lasalvia, A., & Leese, M. (2006). Severe and persistent mental illness: A useful definition for prioritizing community-based mental health service interventions. *Social Psychiatry & Psychiatric Epidemiology, 41*(6), 457–63.

Parikh, S., Segal, Z., Grigoriadis, S., Ravindran, A., Kennedy, S., Lam, R., & Patten, S. B. (2009). Canadian Network for Mood and Anxiety Treatments (CANMAT) Clinical guidelines for the management of major depressive disorder in adults. II. Psychotherapy alone or in combination with antidepressant medication. *Journal of Affective Disorders, 117*, S15–S25.

Park, Y.-J., Kim, H. S., Schwartz-Barcott, D., & Kim, J.-W. (2002). The conceptual structure of hwa-byung in middle-aged Korean women. *Health Care for Women International, 23*, 389–97.

Paris, J. (2008). An evidence-based approach to managing suicidal behavior in patients with BPD. *Social Work in Mental Health, 6*(1–2), 99–108.

———. (2002). Chronic suicidality among patients with borderline personality disorder. *Psychiatric Services, 53*(6), 738–42.

Parker, G., Cheah, Y.-C., & Roy, K. (2001). Do the Chinese somatize depression? A cross-cultural study. *Social Psychiatry & Psychiatric Epidemiology, 36*, 2001.

Perry, A., Tarrier, N., Morriss, R., McCarthy, E., & Limb, K. (1999). Randomised controlled trial of efficacy of teaching patients with bipolar disorder to identify early symptoms of relapse and obtain treatment. *BMJ (Clinical Research Ed.), 318*(7177), 149–53.

Polak, P. R., Kirby, M. W., & Deitchman, W. S. (1995). Treating acutely psychotic patients in private homes. In R. Warner (Ed.), *Alternatives to the hospital for acute psychiatric treatment* (pp. 213–26). Washington, D.C.: American Psychiatric Press.

Pollard, C. A. & Zuercher-White, E. (2003). *The agoraphobia workbook.* Oakland: New Harbinger.

Pope, H. G., Lipinski, J. F., Cohen, B. M., & Axelrod, D. T. (1980). Schizoaffective disorder: An invalid diagnosis? A comparison of schizoaffective disorder, schizophrenia, and affective disorder. *American Journal of Psychiatry, 137*(8), 921–27.

Post, R. M., Leverich, G. S., Altshuler, L. L., Frye, M. A., Suppes, T. M., Keck Jr., P. E., et al. (2003). An overview of recent findings of the Stanley Foundation bipolar network (part I). *Bipolar Disorders, 5*(5), 310.

Power, K., McGoldrick, T., Brown, K., Buchanan, R., Sharp, D., Swanson, V., & Karatzias, A. (2002). A controlled comparison of eye movement desensitization and reprocessing versus exposure plus cognitive restructuring versus waiting list in the treatment of post-traumatic stress disorder. *Clinical Psychology and Psychotherapy, 9*, 299–318.

Pratt, S., & Mueser, K. T. (2002). Social skills training for schizophrenia. In S. Hofmann & M. Tompson (Eds.), *Treating chronic and severe mental disorders: A handbook of empirically supported interventions* (pp. 18–52). New York: Guilford.

Predictors of timely follow-up care among Medicaid-enrolled adults after psychiatric hospitalization (2007). *Psychiatric Services, 58*(12), 1563–69.

Preston, J. (2006). *Integrative brief therapy: Cognitive, psychodynamic, humanistic & neurobehavioral approaches* (2nd ed.). San Luis Obispo, Calif.: Impact.

Prochaska, J. O., & DiClemente, C. C. (1984). *The transtheoretical approach: Crossing the traditional boundaries of therapy.* Malabar, Fla.: Krieger.

Proehl, E. A. (1938). The transition from institutional to social adjustment. *American Sociological Review, 3*(4), 534–40.

Psychosocial interventions. (2005). *Canadian Journal of Psychiatry, 50*, 29S–36S.

Purves, D. & Sands, N. (2009). Crisis and triage clinician's attitudes toward working with people with personality disorder. *Perspectives in Psychiatric Care, 45*(3), 208–15.

Rademaker, A., Vermetten, E., & Kleber, R. (2009). Multimodal exposure-based group treatment for peacekeepers with PTSD: A preliminary evaluation. *Military Psychology, 21*, 482–96.

Randal, P., Simpson, A. I. F., & Laidlaw, T. (2003). Can recovery-focused multi-modal psychotherapy facilitate symptom and function improvement in people with treatment-resistant psychotic illness? A comparison study. *Australian & New Zealand Journal of Psychiatry, 37*(6), 720–27.

Randall, M., & Finkelstein, S. H. (2007). Integration of cognitive behavioral therapy into psychiatric rehabilitation programming. *Psychiatric Rehabilitation Journal, 30*(3), 199–206.

Reding, G., & Raphelson, M. (1995). Around-the-clock mobile psychiatric crisis intervention: Another effective alternative to psychiatric hospitalization. *Community Mental Health Journal, 31*, 179–90.

Resick, P. A., Jordan, C. G., Girelli, S. A., Hutter, C. H., & Marhoefer-Dvorak, S. (1988). A comparative outcome study of behavioral group therapy for sexual assault victims. *Behavior Therapy, 19*, 385–401.

Resick, P. A., & Schnicke, M. K. (1992). Cognitive processing therapy for sexual assault victims. *Journal of Consulting and Clinical Psychology, 60*, 748–56.

Reynolds, S., Wolbert, R., Abney-Cunningham, G., & Patterson, K. (2007). Dialectical therapy for assertive community treatment teams. In M. Linehan, L. Dimeff, & K. Koerner (Eds.), *Dialectical behavior therapy in clinical practice: Applications across disorders and settings* (pp. 298–325). New York: Guilford.

Rogers, S. A., Poey, E. L., Reger, G. M., Tepper, L. & Coleman, E. M. (2002). Religious coping among those with persistent mental illness. *International Journal for the Psychology of Religion, 12*(3), 161–75.

Rohsenow, D. J., Monti, P.M., Martin, R. A., Colby, S. M., Myers, M. G., Gulliver, S. B., Brown, R. A., Mueller, T. I., Gordon, A. & Abrams, D. B. (2004). Motivational enhancement and coping skills training for cocaine abusers: effects on substance use outcomes. *Addiction, 99*, 862–74.

Rooney, K., Hunt, C., Humphreys, L., Harding, D., Mullen, M., & Kearney, J. (2007). Prediction of outcome for veterans with post-traumatic stress disorder using constructs from the transtheoretical model of behavior change. *Australian and New Zealand Journal of Psychiatry, 41*, 590–97.

Rosen, E. J., & Weltman, S. F. (2005). Jewish families: An overview. In M. McGoldrick, J. Giordano, & N. Garcia-Preto (Eds.), *Ethnicity and Family Therapy* (3rd ed., pp. 667–79). New York: Guilford.

Ruggeri, M., Leese M., Thornicroft, G., Bisoffi, G., & Tansella, M. (2000). Definition and prevalence of severe and persistent mental illness. *British Journal of Psychiatry, 177*, 149–55.

Ruggeri, M., Salvi, G., Perwanger, V., Phelan, M., Pellgrini, N., & Parabiaghi, A. (2006). Satisfaction with community and hospital-based emergency services amongst severely mentally ill service users. *Social Psychiatry & Psychiatric Epidemiology, 41*(4), 302–9.

Rumbaut, R. G. (1989). Portraits, patterns, and predictors of the refugee adaptation process. In D. W. haines (Ed.), *Refugees as immigrants: Cambodians, Laotians and Vietnamese in America* (pp. 138–82). Totowa, N.J.: Rowman and Littlefield.

Sachs, G. S., & Gardner-Schuster, E. (2007). Adjunctive treatment of acute mania: A clinical overview. *Acta Psychiatrica Scandinavica, 116*, 27–34.

Sajatovic, M., Davies, M., Bauer, M. S., McBride, L., Hays, R. W., Safavi, R., et al. (2005). Attitudes regarding the collaborative practice model and treatment adherence among individuals with bipolar disorder. *Comprehensive Psychiatry, 46*(4), 272–77.

Satcher, D. (1999). Overview of Cultural Diversity and Mental Health Services. In *Mental Health: A Report of the Surgeon General*. http://www.surgeongeneral.gov/library/mentalhealth/chapter2/sec8.html.

Schnall, E. (2006). Multicultural counseling and the Orthodox Jew. *Journal of Counseling and Development, 84*(3), 276–82.

Schottenbauer, M. A., Glass, C. R., & Arnkoff, D. B. (2005). Outcome research on psychotherapy integration. In J. C. Norcross & M. R. Goldfried (Eds.), *Handbook of psychotherapy integration* (2nd ed., pp. 459–93). New York: Oxford University Press.

Scott, J., Garland, A., & Moorhead, S. (2001). A pilot study of cognitive therapy in bipolar disorders. *Psychological Medicine, 31*(3), 459–67.

Scott, R. (2000). Evaluation of a mobile crisis program: Effectiveness, efficiency, and consumer satisfaction. *Psychiatric Services, 51*(9), 1153–56.

Scurfield, R. M. (1994). War-related trauma: An integrative experiential, cognitive, and spiritual approach. In M. B. Williams & J. F. Sommer, Jr. (Eds.), *Handbook of post-traumatic therapy* (pp. 180–204). Westport, Conn.: Greenwood Press.

Seedat, S., Stein, D., & Carey, P. (2005). Post-traumatic stress disorder in women: Epidemiological and treatment issues. *CNS Drugs, 19*(5), 411–27.

Segal, Z. V., Whitney, D. K., & Lam, R. W. (2001). Clinical guidelines for the treatment of depressive disorders. III. Psychotherapy. *Canadian Journal of Psychiatry, 46,* 29S.

Sensky, T., Turkington, D., Kingdon, D., Scott, J. L., Scott, J., Siddle, R., O'Carroll, M., & Barnes, T. R. E. (2000). A randomized controlled trial of cognitive-behavioral therapy for persistent symptoms in schizophrenia resistant to medication. *Archives of General Psychiatry, 57,* 165–72.

Shalev, A. Y., Friedman, M. J., Foa, E. B., & Keane, T. M. (2000). Integration and summary. In E. Foa, T. Keane, & M. Friedman (Eds.), *Effective treatment of PTSD: Practice guidelines from the International Society for Traumatic Stress Studies* (pp. 359–79). New York: Guilford.

Shapiro, D., & Firth, J. (1987). Prescriptive v. exploratory psychotherapy: Outcomes of the Sheffield Psychotherapy Project. *British Journal of Psychiatry, 151,* 790–99.

Shapiro, D., & Firth-Cozens, J. (1990). Two-year follow-up of the Sheffield Psychotherapy Project. *British Journal of Psychiatry, 157,* 389–91.

Sharpe, L., Tarrier, N., & Rotundo, N. (1994). Treatment of delayed post-traumatic stress disorder following sexual abuse: A case example. *Behavioural and Cognitive Psychotherapy, 22,* 233–42.

Shea, M. T., Elkin, I., Imber, S. D., Sotsky, S. M., Watkins, J. T., Collins, J. F., et al. (1992). Course of depressive symptoms over follow-up: Findings from the National Institute of Mental Health Treatment of Depression Collaborative Research Program. *Archives of General Psychiatry, 49,* 782–87.

Simms, J., McCormack, V., Anderson, R., & Mulholland, C. (2007). Correlates of self-harm behaviour in acutely ill patients with schizophrenia. *Psychology & Psychotherapy: Theory, Research & Practice, 80*(1), 39–49.

Simoneau, T., Miklowitz, D. J., Richards, J. A., Saleem, R., & George, E. L. (1999). Bipolar disorder and family communication: Effects of a psychoeducational treatment program. *Journal of Abnormal Psychology, 108*(4), 588–97.

Skinner, H. A. (1982). The drug abuse screening test. *Addictive Behaviors, 7*(4), 363–71.

Smith, J. (2010). Panic stations: Brief dynamic therapy for panic disorder and generalised anxiety. *Psychodynamic Practice, 16*(1), 25–43.

Soloff, P. H., Lynch, K. G., Kelly, T. M., Malone, K. M., & Mann, J. J. (2000). Characteristics of suicide attempts of patients with major depressive episode and borderline personality disorder: A comparative study. *American Journal of Psychiatry, 157*(4), 601–8.

Stanton, M. D., & Shadish, W. R. (1997). Outcome, attrition, and family-couples treatment for drug abuse: A meta-analysis and review of the controlled, comparative studies. *Psychological Bulletin, 122*(2), 170–91.

Stein, L. I., & Santos, A. B. (1998). *Assertive community treatment of persons with severe mental illness*. New York: Norton.

Stein, L. I., & Test, M. A. (1980). Alternative to mental hospital treatment. I. Conceptual model, treatment program, and clinical evaluation. *Archives of General Psychiatry, 37*(4), 392–97.

Storer, R. M. (2003). A simple cost-benefit analysis of brief interventions on substance abuse at Naval Medical Center Portsmouth. *Military Medicine, 168*(9), 765–68.

Sue, S., Fujino, D.C., Hu, L., & Takeuchi, D. T. (1991). Community mental health services for ethnic minority groups: A test of the cultural responsiveness hypothesis. *Journal of Consulting and Clinical Psychology, 59*, 533–40.

Sue, D. W., & Sue, D. (1999). *Counseling the culturally different*. New York: Wiley.

Swartz, H. A., Markowitz, J. C., & Frank, E. (2002). Interpersonal psychotherapy for unipolar and bipolar disorders. In S. Hofmann &·M. Tompson (Eds.), *Treating chronic and severe mental disorders: A handbook of empirically supported interventions* (pp. 131–58). New York: Guilford.

Swinson, R. P., Soulios, C., Cox, B. J., & Kuch, K. (1992). Brief treatment of emergency room patients with panic attacks. *American Journal of Psychiatry, 149*(7), 944–46.

Szmuckler, G., & Holoway, F. (2001). In-patient treatment. In G. Thornicroft, & Szmuckler (Eds.), *Textbook of community psychiatry* (pp. 265–76). Oxford: Oxford University Press.

Tarrier, N., Barrowclough, C., Haddock, G., & McGovern, J. (1999). The dissemination of innovative cognitive-behavioural psychosocial treatments for schizophrenia. *Journal of Mental Health, 8*(6), 569–82.

Tarrier, N., Beckett, R., Harwood, S., Baker, A., Yusupoff, L., & Ugarteburu, I. (1993). A controlled trial of two cognitive behavioural methods of treating drug-resistant residual psychotic symptoms in schizophrenia patients: I. Outcome. *British Journal of Psychiatry, 162*, 524–32.

Tarrier, N., & Haddock, G. (2002). Cognitive-behavioral therapy for schizophrenia: A case formulation approach. In S. Hofmann & M. Tompson (Eds.), *Treating chronic and severe mental disorders: A handbook of empirically supported interventions* (pp. 69–95). New York: Guilford.

Tarrier, N., Kinney, C., McCarthy, E., Humphreys, L., Wittowski, A., & Morris, J. (2000). Two year follow-up of cognitive behaviour therapy and supportive counseling in the treatment of persistent symptoms in chronic schizophrenia. *Journal of Consulting and Clinical Psychology, 68*, 917–22.

Tarrier, N., Yusupoff, L., Kinney, C., McCarthy, E., Gledhill, A., Haddock, G., & Morris, J. (1998). Randomised controlled trial of intensive cognitive behaviour therapy for patients with chronic schizophrenia. *British Medical Journal, 317*, 303–7.

Teasdale, J. D., Segal, Z. V., Williams, J. M. G., Ridgeway, V. A., Soulsby, J. M., & Lau, M. A. (2000). Prevention of relapse-recurrence in major depression by mindfulness-based cognitive therapy. *Journal of Consulting and Clinical Psychology, 68*, 615–23.

Tennessee opens mental health crisis units. (2007, April 23). *Mental Health* Weekly, *17*(16), 8.

Thombs, D. L. (1999). Introduction to addictive behaviors (2nd ed.). New York: Guilford Press.

Thrasher, S. M., Lovell, K., Noshirvani, M., & Livanou, M. (1996). Cognitive restructuring in the treatment of post-traumatic stress disorder-two single cases. *Clinical Psychology and Psychotherapy, 3*(2), 137–48.

Tibbo, P., Chue, P., & Wright, E. (1999). Hospital outcome measures following assertive community treatment in Edmonton, Alberta. *Canadian Journal of Psychiatry / La Revue Canadienne De Psychiatrie, 44*(3), 276–79.

Tillman, J. G. (2008). A view from Riggs: Treatment resistance and patient authority—IX. Integrative psychodynamic treatment of psychotic disorders. *Journal of the American Academy of Psychoanalysis & Dynamic Psychiatry, 36*(4), 739–61.

Timko, C., DeBenedetti, A., & Billow, R. (2006). Intensive referral to 12-step self-help groups and 6-month substance use disorder outcomes. *Addiction, 101*(5), 678–88.

Tondo, L., Isacsson, G., & Baldessarini, R. J. (2003). Suicidal behaviour in bipolar disorder: Risk and prevention. *CNS Drugs, 17*(7), 491–511.

Torrey, E. F. (1997). *Out of the shadows: Confronting America's mental illness crisis.* New York: Wiley.

Treadwell, K. R. H., Flannery-Schroeder, E. C., & Kendall, P. C. (1995). Ethnic-ity and gender in relation to adaptive functioning, diagnostic status, and treat-ment outcome in children from an anxiety clinic. *Journal of Anxiety Disorders*, *9*, 373–84.

Tsai, J. L., Butcher, J. N., Munoz, R. F., & Vitousek, K. (2004). Culture, ethnicity, and psychopathology. In P. Sutker & H. Adams (Eds.), *Comprehensive hand-book of psychopathology* (3rd ed., pp. 105–27). New York: Springer.

Tsao, J., & Craske, M. (2000). Panic Disorder. In M. Hersen & M. Biaggio (Eds.), *Effective brief therapies: A clinician's guide* (pp. 63–78). San Diego: Academic.

Tseng, W. S., & Hsu, J. (1970). Chinese culture, personality formation and mental illness. *International Journal of Social Psychiatry*, *16*, 5–14.

Tucker, T., Fry, C. L., Lintzeris, N., Baldwin, S., Ritter, A., Donath, S., et al. (2004). Randomized controlled trial of a brief behavioural intervention for reducing hep-atitis C virus risk practices among injecting drug users. *Addiction*, *99*(9), 1157–66.

U.S. Census Bureau (2011a). *Age and sex composition: 2010 Census Briefs*. http://www.census.gov/prod/cen2010/briefs/c2010br-03.pdf.

———. (2011b). *The Hispanic population: 2010 Census Briefs*. http://www.census.gov/prod/cen2010/briefs/c2010br-04.pdf.

U.S. Department of Health and Human Services. (2001). *Mental Health: Culture, Race, and Ethnicity—A Supplement to Mental Health: A Report of the Surgeon General*. Rockville, Md.: U.S. Department of Health and Human Services, Sub-stance Abuse and Mental Health Services Administration, Center for Mental Health Services.

Van Apeldoorn, F. J., Van Hout, W. J. P. J., Mersch, P. P. A., et al. (2008). Is a com-bined therapy more effective than either CBT or SSRI alone? Results of a mul-ticenter trial on panic disorder with or without agoraphobia. *Acta Psychiatrica Scandinavica*, *117*, 260–70.

Van Brunt, D., & Lichstein, K. (2000). Primary Insomnia. In M. Hersen & M. Biaggio (Eds.), *Effective brief therapies: A clinician's guide* (pp. 283–302). San Diego: Academic.

Van Etten, M., & Taylor, S. (1998). Comparative efficacy of treatments for post-traumatic stress disorder: A meta-analysis. *Clinical Psychology and Psychother-apy*, *5*, 126–44.

Virginia Department of Mental Health Mental Retardation and Substance Abuse Services (DMHMRSAS). *2008 mental health law reform*. http://www.dmhmrsas.virginia.gov/OMH-MHReform.htm.

Vittengl, J. R., Clark, L. A., Dunn, T. W., & Jarrett, R. B. (2007). Reducing relapse and recurrence in unipolar depression: A comparative meta-analysis of cognitive-behavioral therapy's effects. *Journal of Consulting and Clinical Psychology*, *75*(3), 475–88.

Vögele, C., Ehlers, A., Meyer, A., Frank, M., Hahlweg, K. & Margraf, J. (2010). Cognitive mediation of clinical improvement after intensive exposure therapy of agoraphobia and social phobia. *Depression and Anxiety*, *27*, 294–301.

Vogl, G., & Zaudig, M. (1985). Investigation of operationalized diagnostic criteria in the diagnosis of schizoaffective and cycloid psychoses. *Comprehensive Psychiatry*, *26*(1), 1–10.

Waddell, M. T., Barlow, D. H., & O'Brien, G. T. (1984). A preliminary investigation of cognitive and relaxation treatment of panic disorder: Effects on intense anxiety vs. "background" anxiety. *Behavior Research and Therapy*, *22*, 393–402.

Warner, R. (1995). *Alternatives to the hospital for acute psychiatric treatment*. Washington, D.C.: American Psychiatric Press.

Watt, M., Stewart, S., Birch, C., & Bernier, D. (2006). Brief CBT for high anxiety sensitivity decreases drinking problems, relief alcohol outcome expectancies, and conformity drinking motives: Evidence from a randomized controlled trial. *Journal of Mental Health*, *15*(6), 683–95.

Westling, B. E., & Öst, L.-G. (1999). Brief cognitive behaviour therapy of panic disorder. *Scandinavian Journal of Behaviour Therapy*, *28*, 49–57.

Westra, H. A., & Dozois, D. J. A. (2006). Preparing clients for cognitive behavioural therapy: A randomized pilot study of motivational interviewing for anxiety. *Cognitive Therapy and Research*, *30*, 481–98.

———. (2008). Integrating motivational interviewing into the treatment of anxiety. In H. Arkowitz, H. A. Westra, W. R. Miller, & S. Rollnick (Eds.), *Motivational interviewing in the treatment of psychological problems* (pp. 26–56). New York: Guilford.

Whaley, A. L. (2002). Symptom clusters in the diagnosis of affective disorder, schizoaffective disorder, and schizophrenia in African Americans. *Journal of the National Medical Association*, *94*(5), 313–19.

White, K. S., & Barlow, D. H. (2002). Panic disorder and agoraphobia. In D. H. Barlow (Ed.), *Anxiety and its disorders: The nature and treatment of anxiety and panic* (2nd ed., pp. 328–79). New York: Guilford.

Wiger, D. E., & Harowski, K. J. (2003). *Essentials of crisis counseling and intervention*. Hoboken, N.J.: Wiley.

Williams, K. E., & Chambless, D. L. (1994). The results of exposure-based treatment in agoraphobia. In S. Friedman (Ed.), *Anxiety disorders in African Americans* (pp. 149–65). New York: Springer.

Williams, M. B. (1994). Establishing safety in survivors of severe sexual abuse. In M. B. Williams & J. F. Sommer, Jr. (Eds.), *Handbook of post-traumatic therapy* (pp. 162–78). Westport, Conn.: Greenwood Press.

Williams, M. B., & Poijula, S. (2002). *The PTSD workbook*. Oakland: New Harbinger Publications.

Wilson, J. P. (1994). The need for an integrative theory of post-traumatic stress disorder. In M. B. Williams & J. F. Sommer, Jr. (Eds.), *Handbook of post-traumatic therapy* (pp. 13–18). Westport, Conn.: Greenwood Press.

Witztum, E., & Buchbinder, J. T. (2001). Strategic culture sensitive therapy with religious Jews. *International Review of Psychiatry, 13*, 117–24.

Wolfe, B. (2005). *Understanding and treating anxiety disorders: An integrative approach to healing the wounded self.* Washington, D.C.: American Psychological Association.

Wolfsdorf, B., & Zlotnik, C. (2001). Affect management in group therapy for women with posttraumatic stress disorder and histories of childhood sexual abuse. *Journal of Clinical Psychology/In Session, 57*(2), 169–81.

Wong, Y. J., Tran, K. K., Kim, S.-H., Van Horne Kerne, V., & Calfa, N. A. (2010). Asian Americans' lay beliefs about depression and professional help seeking. *Journal of Clinical Psychology, 66*(3), 317–32.

Woodward, A. T., Chatters, L. M., Taylor, R. J., Neighbors, H. W., & Jackson, J. S. (2010). Differences in professional and informal help seeking among older African Americans, black Caribbeans, and non-Hispanic whites. *Journal of the Society for Social Work and Research, 1*(3), 124–39.

Woodward, A. T., Taylor, R. J., & Chatters, L. M. (2011). Use of professional and informal support by African American and Black Caribbean men with a mental disorder. *Research on Social Work Practice, 21*(3), 328–36.

Yamamoto, J. (1992). Psychiatric diagnoses and neurasthenia. *Psychiatric Annals, 22*(4), 171–72.

Yatham, L. N., Kennedy, S. H., O'Donovan, C., Parikh, S. V., MacQueen, G., McIntyre, R. S., et al. (2006). Canadian network for mood and anxiety treatments (CANMAT) guidelines for the management of patients with bipolar disorder: Update 2007. *Bipolar Disorders, 8*(6), 721–39.

Ying, Y. (1988). Depressive symptomatology among Chinese-Americans as measured by the CES-D. *Journal of Clinical Psychology, 44*, 739–46.

Young, A. S., Forquer, S. L., Tran, A., Starzynski, M., & Shatkin, J. (2000). Identifying clinical competencies that support rehabilitation and empowerment in individuals with severe and persistent mental illness. *Journal of Behavioral Health Services & Research, 27(3), 321–34.*

Young, J. E., Klosko, J. S., & Weishaar, M. E. (2003). Schema therapy: A practitioner's guide. New York: Guilford.

Zane, N., Sue, S., Chang, J., Huang, L., & Huang, J., et al. (2005). Beyond ethnic match: Effects of client-therapist cognitive match in problem perception, coping orientation, and therapy goals on treatment outcomes. *Journal of Community Psychology, 33(5), 569–85.*

Zaretsky, A. E., Segal, Z. V., & Gemar, M. (1999). Cognitive therapy for bipolar depression: A pilot study. *Canadian Journal of Psychiatry, 44*(5), 491–94.

Zealberg, J., Santos, A., & Fisher, R. (1993). Benefits of mobile crisis programs. *Hospital and Community Psychiatry, 44*, 16–17.

Zerler, H. (2008). Motivational interviewing and suicidality. In H. Arkowitz, H. A. Westra, W. R. Miller, & S. Rollnick (Eds.), *Motivational interviewing in the treatment of psychological problems* (pp. 173–93). New York: Guilford Press.

Zhao, J., & Jin, H. (2010). Effect of antipsychotic medication alone vs. combined with psychosocial intervention on outcomes of early-stage schizophrenia. *Arch Gen Psychiatry, 67*(9), 895–904.

Ziegler, V. E., & Biggs, J. T. (1977). Tricyclic plasma levels. Effect of age, race, sex, and smoking. *Journal of the American Medical Association, 14*, (238), 2167–69.

Zlotnick, C., Shea, T. M., Rosen, K. Simpson, E., Mulrenin, K., Begin, A., & Pearlstein, T. (1997). An affect-management group for women with posttraumatic stress disorder and histories of childhood sexual abuse. *Journal of Traumatic Stress, 10*(3), 425–36.

Zubin, J., & Spring, B. (1977). Vulnerability-A new view of schizophrenia. *Journal of Abnormal Psychology, 86*(2), 103–26.

Zuckoff, A., Swartz, H. A., & Grote, N. K. (2008). Motivational interviewing as a prelude to psychotherapy of depression. In H. Arkowitz, H. A. Westra, W. R. Miller, & S. Rollnick (Eds.), *Motivational interviewing in the treatment of psychological problems* (pp. 109–44). New York: Guilford.

Zuercher-White, E. (1997). *Treating panic disorder and agoraphobia: A step-by-step clinical guide.* Oakland: New Harbinger.

Zuniga, M. (1997). Counseling Mexican American seniors: An overview. *Journal of Multicultural Counseling & Development, 25*(2), 142–55.